THE
GIRLFRIENDS'
GUIDE TO
PREGNANCY
Daily Diary

VICKI IOVINE

POCKET BOOKS

NEW YORK • LONDON • TORONTO • SYDNEY • TOKYO • SINGAPORE

THE AUTHOR OF THIS BOOK IS NOT A PHYSICIAN AND THE IDEAS, PROCEDURES, AND SUGGESTIONS IN THIS BOOK ARE NOT INTENDED AS A SUBSTITUTE FOR THE MEDICAL ADVICE OF A TRAINED HEALTH PROFESSIONAL. ALL MATTERS REGARDING YOUR HEALTH REQUIRE MEDICAL SUPERVISION. CONSULT YOUR PHYSICIAN BEFORE ADOPTING THE SUGGESTIONS IN THIS BOOK, AS WELL AS ABOUT ANY CONDITION THAT MAY REQUIRE DIAGNOSIS OR MEDICAL ATTENTION. THE AUTHOR AND PUBLISHER DISCLAIM ANY LIABILITY ARISING DIRECTLY OR INDIRECTLY FROM THE USE OF THIS BOOK.

AN *Original* PUBLICATION OF POCKET BOOKS

POCKET BOOKS, A DIVISION OF SIMON & SCHUSTER INC.
1230 AVENUE OF THE AMERICAS, NEW YORK, NY 10020

ISBN: 0–671–00290–2

FIRST POCKET BOOKS TRADE PAPERBACK PRINTING NOVEMBER 1996

10 9 8 7 6 5 4 3 2 1

POCKET AND COLOPHON ARE REGISTERED TRADEMARKS OF SIMON & SCHUSTER INC.

COVER AND INTERIOR DESIGN AND INTERIOR ILLUSTRATIONS BY LESLEY EHLERS
FRONT COVER ILLUSTRATIONS BY GARY JOHNSON

PRINTED IN THE U.S.A.

FOR ORDERS OTHER THAN BY INDIVIDUAL CONSUMERS, POCKET BOOKS GRANTS A DISCOUNT ON THE PURCHASE OF 10 OR MORE COPIES OF SINGLE TITLES FOR SPECIAL MARKETS OR PREMIUM USE. FOR FURTHER DETAILS, PLEASE WRITE TO THE VICE-PRESIDENT OF SPECIAL MARKETS, POCKET BOOKS, 1633 BROADWAY, NEW YORK, NY 10019-6785, 8TH FLOOR.

FOR INFORMATION ON HOW INDIVIDUAL CONSUMERS CAN PLACE ORDERS, PLEASE WRITE TO MAIL ORDER DEPARTMENT, SIMON & SCHUSTER INC., 200 OLD TAPPAN ROAD, OLD TAPPAN, NJ 07675.

DEDICATED WITH LOVE

To GramAndrea, who forced me to take
typing in high school, but who still types faster than I do.
Thanks for overlooking some of my exaggerations, for
loving our kids, and for working as hard as
I did to meet my deadline.

—— AND ——

To Jody, who became every aspect of me except author
so that I could work without being noticeably absent,
and who has such a powerful smile that you can
feel it as well as see it.

INTRODUCTION

Never has a day been more anxiously anticipated than the birth of your baby. As a kid, you probably thought there were several light-years between holidays. Getting your driver's license felt like it took forever to finally happen, as did your graduation, your twenty-first birthday and maybe even your engagement. Small potatoes next to the journey of a woman who has gone from missing her period to becoming the mother of a child.

Every day for the next year will be surprising, confusing, thrilling, tedious, nerve-racking and hopefully not too nauseating, but you are not alone because *The Girlfriends' Guide to Pregnancy Daily Diary* is here for you all the way, and we won't desert you postpartum.

You'll learn quickly that the greatest myth of pregnancy is that it lasts nine months. Average gestation is forty weeks, which even with this new math stuff sounds like ten months to us.

The Diary is organized to be appropriate to your transformation through all four trimesters of pregnancy: the three when the baby is inside of you, and the fourth, when you're still in a pregnant state but the baby is outside of you. Snippets of information, suggestions for coping, top ten lists and some good belly laughs are given in daily doses, keeping in mind the pregnancy rules of thumb regarding information: "Don't give us more than we can handle at any given time," or "If you tell us too much, we'll just forget it anyway."

Keep some notes, mark some milestones, record information from doctors' visits, but most of all, truly enjoy this time because, in the end, it's over before you know it.

TOP **10** GREATEST LIES ABOUT PREGNANCY

10. LAMAZE WORKS.

9. MORNING SICKNESS IS GONE BY LUNCHTIME.

8. MATERNITY CLOTHES ARE SO MUCH CUTER NOW.

7. YOU WILL HAVE YOUR PREPREGNANCY FIGURE BACK IN THREE MONTHS, ESPECIALLY IF YOU NURSE.

6. OIL MASSAGES PREVENT STRETCH MARKS.

5. PREGNANT WOMEN HAVE THE MOST BEAUTIFUL SKIN AND HAIR.

4. "I SWEAR, YOUR FACE HASN'T CHANGED AT ALL!"

3. PREGNANCY BRINGS A MAN AND WOMAN CLOSER TOGETHER (YEAH, YOU AND YOUR OBSTETRICIAN!).

2. "YOU HAVEN'T GOTTEN BIG ANYWHERE BUT YOUR BELLY!"

1. PREGNANCY ONLY LASTS NINE MONTHS.

FIRST TRIMESTER

9-12-96
....
D A T E

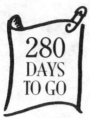

280
DAYS
TO GO

Yippee! You are going to have a baby!
Welcome to the sorority of mothers. There is
nothing the world loves more than a pregnant
woman. The countdown begins as you embark on
what remains of the approximately 280 days it
takes to cook a baby.

Now, mark the date of your last period on this
page, since that's how medical people measure how
pregnant you are. In other words, you may already
be four or even six weeks pregnant. Think about it,
you already have at least a month under your belt,
so to speak, and it was a piece of cake...
only nine more to go.

N O T E S:..
....
....
....
....
....

9-21-96

D A T E

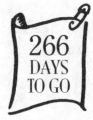

266
DAYS
TO GO

Mark here the date
of conception.
You may know when "it" happened
through good old-fashioned intuition,
or you can count 14 days after your
last period and mark that as
the Big Event.
A few juicy details wouldn't hurt...
you know how nosy we
Girlfriends can be.

N O T E S: a 2 days after

FIRST TRIMESTER

10-9-96
_____

D A T E

252
DAYS
TO GO

Congratulations...again!!! Now that
we know you're pregnant, let's begin
the countdown. For consistency's sake,
let's assume you took the pregnancy test
on the day your always-dependable-28-day-cycle
period was supposed to start. And, to
complete the fantasy, let's pretend
that day was today.

Mark this page with today's date.

N O T E S : 23 day cycle. - so I knew
I was pregnant dr 10-5 and confirmed
10-6. A funny story - I didn't
believe it and went back to bed
before reading the test accurately.
Then, shock 4 hrs later. ☺

FIRST TRIMESTER

251
DAYS
TO GO

Are you still comatose, or have you leapt into
that hyperactive glee of someone with a huge
secret to share? Normal reactions to positive
pregnancy test results span a spectrum of emotions
from absolute terror, through dazed ambivalence,
to euphoria, so don't second-guess your
feelings. In fact, do yourself a favor and
try out all the possible emotions just to get
the full pregnancy experience.

Mark today's date on this page, and
tomorrow's date on the next page, and so on.
There, now we've got the rhythm.

N O T E S:...

....

....

....

....

....

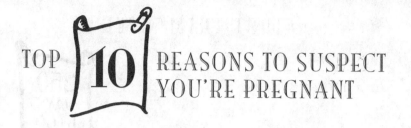

TOP **10** REASONS TO SUSPECT YOU'RE PREGNANT

10. YOUR BREASTS ARE BIGGER, PUFFIER AND A LOT MORE SENSITIVE.

9. YOU NEED TO URINATE FREQUENTLY, ESPECIALLY IN THE MIDDLE OF THE NIGHT.

8. YOU'RE EVEN MORE EXHAUSTED THAN USUAL.

7. PHANTOM MENSTRUAL CRAMPS—YOU SWEAR YOUR PERIOD IS ABOUT TO START.

6. YOU'RE DIZZY AND LIGHT-HEADED, AND YOU MAY EVEN FAINT.

5. NAUSEOUS? WE'RE TALKING, MORNING, NOON AND NIGHT SICKNESS.

4. THE WORLD BEGINS TO SMELL STRANGE AND YOU THINK YOU COULD FREELANCE WITH POLICE DOGS TO SNIFF OUT ILLEGAL SUBSTANCES.

3. FEEL LIKE YOU'RE LOSING YOUR MIND OR CONTROL OF YOUR EMOTIONS? WELCOME TO PREGNANCY INSANITY.

2. YOU MAY THINK NO PERIOD IS A TELLTALE SIGN, THOUGH FOR YOU IRREGULAR GALS, IT'S OFTEN NOT YOUR FIRST CLUE.

1. WORLD-FAMOUS WOMEN'S INTUITION. MANY WOMEN SWEAR THEY KNEW THE MOMENT OF CONCEPTION.

FIRST TRIMESTER

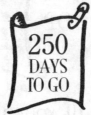

250
DAYS
TO GO

Pregnancy Test

If it wasn't your doctor who performed
your pregnancy test, then today is the day you
should call and make an appointment
(if you haven't already). Most women can take
a dozen home pregnancy tests, line them up
on the bathroom counter and read all positive
results and still not consider themselves
officially pregnant until someone in an office
with a plastic model of a uterus on
display tells them it is so.

NOTES:

FIRST TRIMESTER

249 DAYS TO GO

Almost all husbands ask the same ridiculous question when their mates announce they are pregnant. "Are you sure?"

They don't mean to challenge your ability to understand the instructions "blue, pregnant; white, not pregnant." It's just that they want you to make it clear for them that they have, indeed, been tagged "it" and there are no "backsies."

Be honest, you felt the same way, too, when you first learned the news.

NOTES:..

....

....

....

....

....

FIRST TRIMESTER

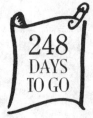

248
DAYS
TO GO

So, exactly how long is this going to last?
The average pregnancy is anywhere from
240 to 300 days, with most people
accepting 280 as the norm. Slightly more
women give birth before the full
280 days than after, but only 5 percent
actually deliver the goods on their due date.

N O T E S: ....

....

....

....

....

....

10-14
DATE

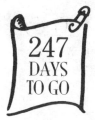

247
DAYS
TO GO

Here's a little math to keep your addled
mind in shape. To calculate your due date,
count back three months from the first day
of your last period, then add seven days to
that number. Oh, never mind, ask your
doctor to figure it out for you.
It's never accurate anyway.

NOTES:

..........10-15..........
DATE

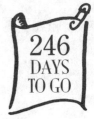

246
DAYS
TO GO

Prepare to become a "precious vessel" for
the next nine (ten) months. People just love
pregnant women. They will want to protect and
encourage you. They will also want to give
you unsolicited advice and subject you to endless
stories about their own pregnancies, or any other
pregnancy they have heard of. Practice smiling
and silently make lists of potential
baby names while they prattle on.

NOTES: ....
....
....
....
....
....

245
DAYS
TO GO

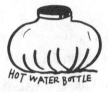

HOT WATER BOTTLE

It's common to get menstrual cramps during the first few weeks of your pregnancy.
It doesn't mean you're getting your period, simply that your uterus is getting adjusted to its new job. Don't worry about the cramps if they are fairly mild and not accompanied by bleeding, because they do not signify any danger to the pregnancy. You are fine...just another victim of nature's practical jokes.

N O T E S:..
....
....
....
....
....

TOP 10 GREATEST CONCERNS OF PREGNANT WOMEN

10. WILL MY BREASTS STAY THIS BIG FOREVER? (PLEASE, GOD!)

9. WILL I FEEL THIS SICK AND TIRED FOR THE ENTIRE NINE (TEN) MONTHS?

8. WILL MY HUSBAND EVER REALLY UNDERSTAND WHAT I AM GOING THROUGH?

7. WILL IT HURT TO DELIVER THE BABY?

6. HOW BADLY WILL IT HURT TO DELIVER THE BABY?

5. WILL IT HURT MORE THAN A BIKINI WAX? LESS THAN A BROKEN LEG?

4. WILL I GET ALL UGLY AND FAT?

3. WILL EVERYTHING DOWN THERE SHRINK BACK TO NORMAL AFTER THE BABY IS BORN?

2. WILL I BE A GOOD MOTHER?

1. WILL THE BABY BE OK?

244
DAYS
TO GO

Stop torturing yourself because you had a couple of drinks, were on medication or addicted to diet sodas before you realized you were pregnant. If only people who were vice-free had babies, there would be no such thing as rock and roll.

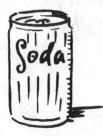

Talk to your doctor about your concerns...doctors are never as scandalized as you think they'll be. The baby will be fine, but do clean up your act now since it's not nice to be selfish.

N O T E S: ....
....
....
....
....
....

FIRST TRIMESTER

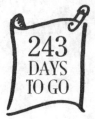

243 DAYS TO GO

Morning sickness does not usually
begin its siege the minute you pass the
pregnancy test. It lulls you into a false sense
of security and then strikes right when you
are certain you have avoided nausea completely.
So don't start the self-congratulating yet,
because it still might rear its ugly head.

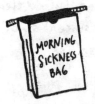

MORNING
SICKNESS
BAG

NOTES: ....
....
....
....
....
....

10-19
DATE

242
DAYS
TO GO

Isn't it scary how devoted you already
feel to this pregnancy? Just a few days ago,
you were obliviously living your life,
unaware of your little passenger.
You might not have even been trying
to get pregnant. And now your entire
consciousness is devoted to staying pregnant.
They really get a hold on us early.

NOTES:..
....
....
....
....
....

FIRST TRIMESTER

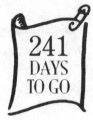

241
DAYS
TO GO

Sit down because I have something unbelievable
to tell you. Right about now your baby's heart
will begin to beat. Think about it...
there is a little human inside of you! It will
be a few more weeks before the doctor can
let you hear the heartbeat, but by next week,
you can see the heartbeat with an
ultrasound. It looks like a lima bean with
a flickering light inside.

N O T E S: ....
....
....
....
....
....

FIRST TRIMESTER

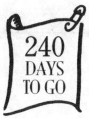

240
DAYS
TO GO

Feeling a bit haggard, Girlfriend? Perhaps it's because your bladder has turned against you. This mutinous organ seems to wake you up every time you settle into a nice dream state. Try to outsmart it...don't drink fluids after dinner. This will help a little, but the only real cure is the passage of time. This urgency to peepee passes as the progesterone levels out. Trouble is, it comes back again in the third trimester when your bladder is little more than a fetal trampoline.

N O T E S:...
....
....
....
....
....

FIRST TRIMESTER

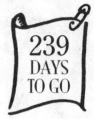

239
DAYS
TO GO

Do you feel addle-brained yet?
A constant state of confusion
and distraction defines the mental
health of pregnant women.
You get so involved with what's going
on inside you that at times, the outside
world is little more than an intrusion.

N O T E S: ....
....
....
....
....
....

10 · 23

D A T E

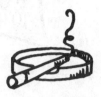

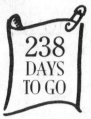

238
DAYS
TO GO

Rarely do we Girlfriends preach, and we
generally loathe it when people do it to us.
But here is our one exception.
YOU MUST STOP SMOKING NOW.
It's not just bad for your pregnancy, but we
know that if you smoke now, you are
almost certain to smoke after the baby is
born, and that is akin to raising your child
in a subway station, as far as we're concerned.
Don't be embarrassed, you probably haven't done
any damage to your baby (after all, many of our
own mothers smoked when pregnant with us),
but you will if this habit persists.

N O T E S: ....
....
....
....
....
....

FIRST TRIMESTER

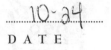
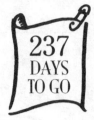
Spend your lunch hour at a bookstore
(preferably one that allows you to eat and browse
at the same time). Look at all the books about
pregnancy. Then immediately disregard all
those written by people who have never given birth.
Among the two or three that are left, toss out
those that have any scary parts. Now,
proceed to the counter and buy
The Girlfriends' Guide to Pregnancy.

NOTES: ....

....

....

....

....

FIRST TRIMESTER

<u>10-25</u>
DATE

236
DAYS
TO GO

It's never too early to check out your
insurance policy to see what
pregnancy procedures are covered
and how long it will pay for you
and the baby to recover in the
hospital after delivery. Call and speak to
the insurers to clarify anything you don't
understand, and then get their names
so that you can blame them later.
Come to think of it, this is a good job
for your husband.

NOTES:..
....
....
....
....
....

FIRST TRIMESTER

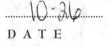

235
DAYS
TO GO

Spend some time today calling Girlfriends who
have had babies in your area and asking them
about their obstetricians. You may want to stay
with the gynecologist who fitted your diaphragm;
then again, you may want to begin interviewing
doctors to find someone who shares your
childbirth vision and understands your particular
little needs, such as his willingness to take your
call immediately when you can't figure out
where the hair that is sprouting out of
your nipple came from.

N O T E S : ....

....

....

....

....

....

FIRST TRIMESTER

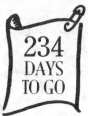

234
DAYS
TO GO

The best way to find an
obstetrician is the same way
we find hairdressers, plastic surgeons and stores
selling Snackwells half-price; we ask
our Girlfriends. Sure, the AMA has its listings,
and your general practitioner can refer you to
someone, but the real skinny comes from someone
who has actually launched a baby into the hands
of that doctor and lived to tell about it.

N O T E S : ....
....
....
....
....
....

10-28
DATE

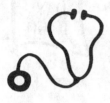

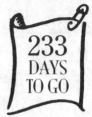

233
DAYS
TO GO

A major consideration in choosing obstetricians
is learning what hospital they are affiliated with.
This can be particularly crucial in larger cities,
where there are several hospitals in which babies
are delivered. Does the hospital your potential
doctor works in have a neonatal intensive care unit
should you need it? What are the birthing rooms
like? How far is the drive from your home?
Most critical of all, does this hospital have a
full-time anesthesiologist so you won't be
calling out in vain for pain relief at 4 A.M.?

NOTES:

...10-29........
DATE

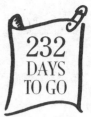

232
DAYS
TO GO

Are you hoping for a boy or a girl?
I'm not talking about your baby; I mean
your obstetrician. While there are still
significantly more men in this practice,
there are thousands of women, too, and
you may just find yourself more comfortable
being looked after by someone who was born
with a uterus. As one Girlfriend asked,
"Would you hire a mechanic who had never
even driven a car before?"

NOTES: ....
....
....
....
....
....

10-30
....

D A T E

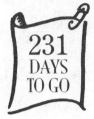

231 DAYS TO GO

Remember, morning sickness is
arbitrary, like being picked for jury duty.
It is no reflection on how well you are
doing this pregnancy.

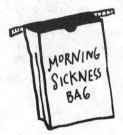

N O T E S : ....
....
....
....
....
....

FIRST TRIMESTER

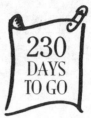

230
DAYS
TO GO

If this is your second or subsequent
pregnancy, you will notice that you
already look pregnant. Those taut little
stomach muscles were permanently traumatized
by your first pregnancy, and they let go
as soon as they got the news
about the new baby.

N O T E S: ....
....
....
....
....
....

FIRST TRIMESTER

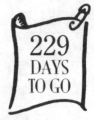

229
DAYS
TO GO

No matter how urgent your need to
express yourself, try to sound calm
when reminding your mate that
your luscious new breasts are to be admired
from afar for a few more weeks.
Husbands are jumpy as it is, and they get
worse after having been slapped
a couple of times when they reached
for their new "toys."

N O T E S : ....

....

....

....

....

....

TOP **10** COMMANDMENTS OF MORNING SICKNESS

10. EAT SMALL AMOUNTS OF BLAND FOODS ALL DAY LONG.

9. DON'T EAT ANYTHING THAT DOESN'T SMELL APPEALING TO YOU.

8. EAT SOMETHING AROUND 4 A.M. , OR AFTER YOUR LAST MIDDLE-OF-THE-NIGHT VISIT TO THE TOILET.

7. TAKE YOUR PRENATAL VITAMINS AT NIGHT, OR STOP ALTOGETHER UNTIL YOU ARE FEELING BETTER. (YOUR DOCTOR MAY WANT YOU TO TAKE FOLIC ACID SUPPLEMENTS IN THE MEANTIME.)

6. DO NOT TAKE YOUR VITAMINS WITH CITRUS JUICE.

5. WHEN NOTHING SOUNDS APPETIZING, TRY A BOWL OF CEREAL WITH MILK, OR A PIECE OF SWEET FRUIT.

4. IF THE THOUGHT OF CHEWING ANY KIND OF FOOD MAKES YOU SICK, TRY SUCKING ON NATURAL LICORICE DROPS.

3. TRY WEARING THE ELASTIC WRISTBANDS THAT ARE SOLD IN PHARMACIES TO PREVENT SEASICKNESS.

2. SKIP THE SALTINES UNLESS YOU HAVE A REAL CRAVING FOR THEM (WHICH I CAN'T IMAGINE UNLESS YOU ARE A PARROT).

1. FOLLOW YOUR CRAVINGS. IF YOU REALLY WANT SOME PARTICULAR TYPE OF FOOD, THERE IS A GOOD CHANCE IT WILL ACTUALLY MAKE YOU FEEL A LITTLE BETTER IF YOU EAT IT.

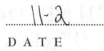

11-2

DATE

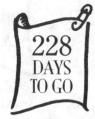

228
DAYS
TO GO

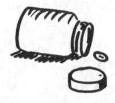

Prenatal vitamins are the size of Scud missiles.
I swear I have seen cellular phones that are
smaller. If you have trouble swallowing yours
without gagging during this trimester of what
might seem like constant gagging, try washing
them down with something tastier than water.
Chocolate milk can be nice; after all, you do need
the calcium. Just don't take prenatals with citrus
juice since the acid can make them even more
offensive to your sensitive stomach.

NOTES: ....
....
....
....
....
....

FIRST TRIMESTER

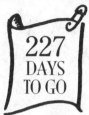

227
DAYS
TO GO

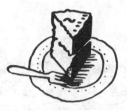

Let's talk about food. The Girlfriends'
rule of thumb is this: Don't eat anything that
makes your stomach lurch just because some dumb
book says that you should. And don't deny yourself
an ice cream cone every now and then, if that's
what you have your chubby little heart set on.
Moderation in everything, Girlfriend, except
maybe self-congratulations, which you should be
showering on yourself.

N O T E S:...
....
....
....
....
....

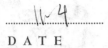

D A T E

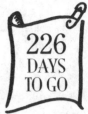

226
DAYS
TO GO

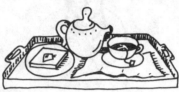

Become friends with the morning talk shows.
It really helps to combat morning sickness
if you take fifteen to twenty minutes to get
out of bed in the morning (of course, it helps
even more not to get out of bed at all,
but we're dreamin' here). Breakfast in bed
is even better, so sweetly suggest to your mate
that a little toast and tea would be
tremendously appreciated.

N O T E S: ....
....
....
....
....
....

FIRST TRIMESTER

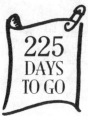

225
DAYS
TO GO

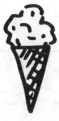

Some men get morning sickness and
food cravings to keep their pregnant wives
company. Yeah, right! If yours does, firmly
remind him that there is only room for
one heifer in this corral, pardner.
No Braxton Hicks contractions? No rewards
of Rocky Road in a sugar cone.

NOTES: ....
....
....
....
....
....

FIRST TRIMESTER

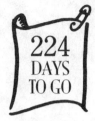

224 DAYS TO GO

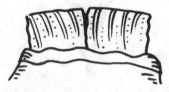

Stand up slowly! Many gestating women
experience light-headedness and dizziness
because pregnancy has lowered their
blood pressure. Getting out of bed can be
particularly disorienting (isn't it always?),
so give yourself plenty of time to
work into a standing position. Two or three
hours sounds about right, doesn't it?

N O T E S: ....
....
....
....
....
....

FIRST TRIMESTER

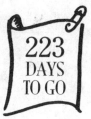

223 DAYS TO GO

Food cravings are real and should be indulged. Begin to trust your instincts in this pregnancy/motherhood area, even if you end up eating nectarines four times a day for three weeks straight. It may not be that your body has a natural, infallible nutrition gauge, but it does instinctively know what it can eat without vomiting.

NOTES:...
....
....
....
....
....

.........11-8.........
DATE

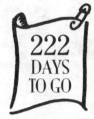

222
DAYS
TO GO

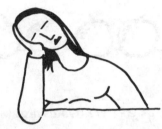

Naps are completely appropriate during
this time, be they in bed, at your desk, or
on the copier room floor. Just make sure
you aren't lying on any important documents
or precious fabrics, because pregnant
nappers tend to drool.

NOTES: ....
....
....
....
....
....

FIRST TRIMESTER

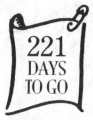

221
DAYS
TO GO

Take a closer look in the mirror after your
shower this morning. See how brown your
nipples look? How about all those blue veins
running like road maps over your breasts?
Yes, pregnancy is a total body experience.

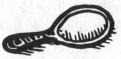

NOTES: ....
....
....
....
....
....

FIRST TRIMESTER

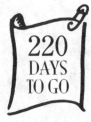

220 DAYS TO GO

Do you have more headaches these days? Let's see, why could that be? Your hormones are at a toxic level, you aren't getting enough sleep, you've gone cold turkey on caffeine and diet sodas and you are a little distracted by your impending motherhood. Knock yourself out and take a Tylenol, but remember to ask your doctor first (God, we're conscientious)! If this is your biggest transgression in ten months, you must be a close personal friend of Mother Teresa.

N O T E S: ....

....

....

....

....

....

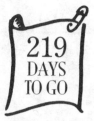

219
DAYS
TO GO

Are ordinary smells beginning to offend you?
Join the sorority and give the cat feeding and litter
box jobs to your mate. Keep the windows wide
open, especially in the car, whenever weather
permits. It's also a good idea to stay out of all
delicatessens and the dairy section of your grocery
store. Don't trust your nose implicitly, however.
Always get a second opinion from a
non-gestater before throwing an
entire meat loaf down the
garbage disposal.

CAT

NOTES: ....
....
....
....
....
....

11-12
....
DATE

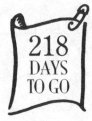

218
DAYS
TO GO

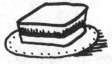

Having a hard time eating foods from
all the major food groups? Don't fret...
many pregnant women can live on little more
than grilled cheese sandwiches on white bread
for days on end. Go easy on yourself and
avoid all foods that make your eyes water;
you and the baby will still thrive.
You'll make up for it in a couple of weeks.

NOTES: ....
....
....
....
....
....

11·13

DATE

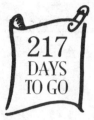

217
DAYS
TO GO

You will be up anyway at 4 or 5 A.M.
going to the bathroom, so take an
extra minute to eat a bowl of cereal or a
piece of bread before you go back to sleep.
A full stomach when you wake up to begin your
day can minimize rise-and-shine retching.

NOTES:..
....
....
....
....
....

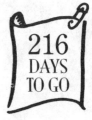

216 DAYS TO GO

Treat yourself to one of those books that
show photos of babies as they grow in the uterus.
Skip any of the scary or preachy text, but
find the pictures because they are miraculous.

I still can't figure out how they got the
camera in there!

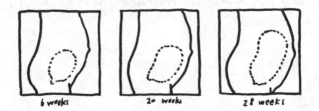

6 weeks   20 weeks   28 weeks

N O T E S: ....
....
....
....
....
....

FIRST TRIMESTER

215
DAYS
TO GO

Want to change your mind about the
motherhood business? On second thought, does
this 280 days of growing big as a hippo
(an adorable hippo, of course) and delivering
a baby out of your dainty little privates appall
more than thrill you? Every honest
Girlfriend will admit to times of wanting to
escape her pregnancy. Don't worry, this is
just a sign of your superior intelligence in
considering the full nature of the task
you have undertaken.

NOTES:

FIRST TRIMESTER

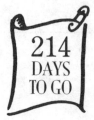

214
DAYS
TO GO

Now that you are pregnant, do you find that
you adore all babies? If the answer is no,
don't worry your pretty little head one minute. I
can say, with total certainty, that your own
little baby will be much prettier, quieter,
cleaner and generally superior to the
garden-variety babies you see in public.
I know mine were.

NOTES: ....
....
....
....
....
....

FIRST TRIMESTER

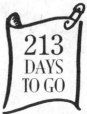

213
DAYS
TO GO

Guess what...your husband is pregnant, too!
And he may be having a hard time digesting
the fact that, even though he has the emotional
inner life of a fifteen-year-old, he is turning
into Ward Cleaver. Don't be surprised if he
takes on some of your pregnancy symptoms.
If you sleep a lot, he may, too. If you crave
raspberry sorbet, he may, too. If you feel
nauseous, he may, too. Try to be tolerant,
but feel free to draw the line if he also gets gas.

NOTES:..
....
....
....
....
....

FIRST TRIMESTER

212
DAYS
TO GO

Not feeling like your usual sexy thing?
What with nausea, sore breasts and fatigue,
most "breeders" like you couldn't care less
about shaving their legs and slipping on the
black stockings. In fact, getting your teeth
brushed might be the most attention you have
paid to your appearance in days. Don't worry,
Girlfriend. Rent your husband a sexy video
(you can nap during it) and wait a few more
weeks because the second trimester just may
unleash the sex goddess in you.

NOTES:...
....
....
....
....
....

TOP 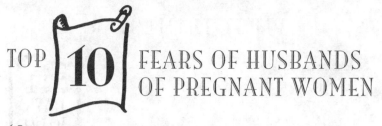 FEARS OF HUSBANDS OF PREGNANT WOMEN

10. HE WILL BE FORCED TO CUT THE UMBILICAL CORD.

9. HE WILL FAINT DURING DELIVERY (OR WORSE YET, HE WILL STAY CONSCIOUS AND HAVE TO WATCH THE WHOLE THING).

8. HE WILL NEVER BE ABLE TO HAVE SEX WITH HIS WIFE AGAIN AFTER SEEING HIS FAVORITE PLAYGROUND BULLDOZED BY A BABY'S GIGANTIC HEAD.

7. HE WILL BE AS BAD/GOOD A FATHER AS HIS OWN FATHER WAS.

6. HE WILL BE BOUND TO YOU, A WEEPY, JUMPY, GASSY, OVERWEIGHT SHADOW OF HIS FORMER SWEETHEART, FOR THE REST OF HIS LIFE.

5. HE WILL HAVE TO DELIVER THE BABY HIMSELF.

4. HE WILL NOT BE ABLE TO AFFORD THE BABY. (HE MAY HAVE A POINT HERE, BUT DON'T ENCOURAGE HIM.)

3. YOU WILL DIE OR RUN OFF AND LEAVE HIM WITH A TINY STRANGER TO CARE FOR.

2. HE WILL BARF DURING DELIVERY AND YOU'LL REPEAT THE TALE FOR THE NEXT TWENTY-FIVE YEARS.

1. IF HE BECOMES A FATHER, HE CANNOT BE THE BABY ANYMORE.

FIRST TRIMESTER

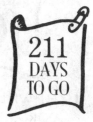

211
DAYS
TO GO

It is very common for fathers-to-be to
feel frightened to have sex with their
pregnant mates. Apparently, they worry that
they will hurt the baby. Isn't it just like a
man to automatically overestimate the
penetrative powers of his penis? It's up to
you how you handle this. If you're feeling
amorous, explain that the baby is completely
protected. If you crave celibacy,
congratulate him on his "huge" sacrifice.

N O T E S : ....
....
....
....
....
....

FIRST TRIMESTER

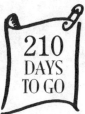

Have you told your father that you're
going to have a baby? Think about it...
this is the first time the two of you have
actually acknowledged that you are no longer
a virgin. If this feels a little bit weird, just
wait until you pull out a giant breast
and start nursing in front of him.
Close Encounters of the Freudian Kind.

NOTES:..
....
....
....
....
....

FIRST TRIMESTER

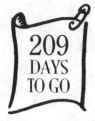

209
DAYS
TO GO

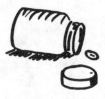

Your doctor has probably prescribed prenatal
vitamins. Do us all a favor and don't start
adding other vitamin or mineral supplements
on the eager-beaver theory that if a little is good,
a lot is better. The same logic that has you
giving up caffeine and aspirin applies to
all that stuff on the shelves in the health
food store, too....no matter what your
sister's yoga teacher says.

N O T E S: ....
....
....
....
....
....

FIRST TRIMESTER

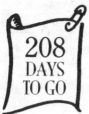
208
DAYS
TO GO

Most mommy Girlfriends have the
compassion not to repeat labor and delivery
horror stories to pregnancy virgins
(hey, good oxymoron!). They wait until
you have stories of your own before going
into contraction-by-contraction detail
of their ordeals.

If someone just can't bear to wait to share
tales of endless labors and stitches from
stem to stern, you are completely
within your rights to stop her. Kindly explain
that you want to be "surprised."

N O T E S:...
....
....
....
....
....

........11:23........
D A T E

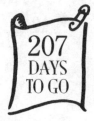

207
DAYS
TO GO

Talk about understatement! Most pregnancy
books warn that you may experience some
"moodiness" at this special time.
Moody, schmoody. Welcome to the madhouse!

Have you found yourself screeching because your
mate brought you vanilla ice cream when you
clearly asked for chocolate, which only goes to
prove that he never listens to you since you clearly
said chocolate, and if he ever paid attention he
would know by now that you never eat vanilla...
in fact, you loathe vanilla...and if he doesn't
care enough about the baby....
Never mind, hand over the ice cream!

N ON O T E S:..
....
....
....
....
....

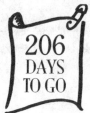

206 DAYS TO GO

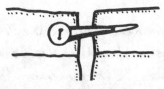

Pants won't button all the way to the top?
Well, you know what they say, the
waistline is the first thing to go.

Here's a trick: Take a hair elastic, hook it around
the top button, run it through the opposing hole,
and then back around the button. There, isn't that
a little more comfortable? No one knows but us,
and we'll never tell. A perfect time to acknowledge
you should no longer be tucking in tops.

N O T E S :..
....
....
....
....
....

FIRST TRIMESTER

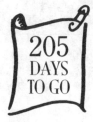

205
DAYS
TO GO

While I have never believed the PMS insanity defense, I must confess that I can see its value for pregnant women. Between memory lapse, distorted judgment and unbearable sensitivity, we can make Sybil look composed.

Suffice it to say, this is not the best time to sign any binding legal documents, operate heavy machinery or change your hairstyle.

N O T E S: ....

....

....

....

....

....

11·26

D A T E

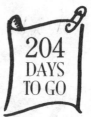

204
DAYS
TO GO

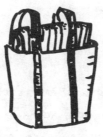

Keep big old towels in the front seat of your
car so that you have something to barf
into if the urge should strike while you are stuck
in traffic. One of the most charming aspects
of morning sickness is its refusal to limit
itself to those hours before noon or to
respect simulated leather interiors.

N O T E S : ....
....
....
....
....
....

FIRST TRIMESTER

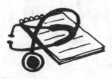

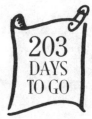

203 DAYS TO GO

Don't be afraid to ask your doctor the questions that really concern you, no matter how ridiculous. First of all, your insurance is probably paying big bucks for this privilege. Second, doctors forget how truly uninformed first-timers really are. Remember, no matter how often you may think about your doctor, doctors only think about you while you are sitting (or lying) right in their faces. No matter how compelling we find ourselves, doctors don't waste their time telling other doctors about the new stooge in their practice.

N O T E S: ....
....
....
....
....
....

FIRST TRIMESTER

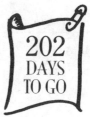

202
DAYS
TO GO

Don't take it personally if your husband seems less enthusiastic about your pregnancy than you. His breasts don't hurt, he's not worried about getting the baby out of his body and he certainly isn't crying every time he sees a diaper commercial on TV. It's just not real to him yet.

It turns out that there is absolutely no correlation between a man who is enchanted by his wife's pregnancy and a man who will eventually sacrifice every Saturday morning coaching Little League.

N O T E S :..

....

....

....

....

....

11:29
DATE

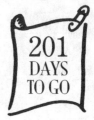

201
DAYS
TO GO

Try sucking on licorice drops to soothe a
choppy stomach. If you hate licorice,
try other hard candies. Fruit-flavored Popsicles
can do wonders, too. Sure, you are completely
ignoring the champion foods like liver and
broccoli, but what's the use of going to
the effort of chewing them if you're just
going to barf them right up?

NOTES:...
....
....
....
....
....

FIRST TRIMESTER

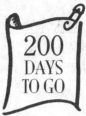

200
DAYS
TO GO

No pregnancy is fully experienced without
the mommy dissolving into tears for no
reason at least three or four times. It can be
the sound of a lullaby, the sight of your own
baby pictures when your own parents looked
so young and optimistic or it might be an
imagined slight such as no one offering you a seat
on the bus. Once the floodgates are open, they
are difficult to close again. You might start out
crying about one thing…then continue to cry
about something completely unrelated.

Lie down and apply cool compresses.

N O T E S:..
....
....
....
....
....

FIRST TRIMESTER

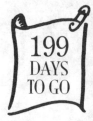

199
DAYS
TO GO

Meet a new pregnant woman today. Gestation is so much more fun when you share it with someone who completely relates to your concerns and shares your obsession with all things baby.

Expectant moms are easy to meet because you already have so much in common. Talk to other women in the o.b.'s waiting room or the supermarket. A good icebreaker is, "So, when are you due?" After that, they will have to pry you apart.

NOTES: ....
....
....
....
....
....

12-2
D A T E

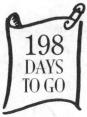

198
DAYS
TO GO

Have you begun fretting about how much
or how little (less likely, but it happens)
weight you have gained? This is a universal
thorn in the ample sides of pregnant women.
Stop comparing yourself to standards in
unenlightened books...or, worse, soap
opera stars, who swear they work up to
their due dates and give birth in their dressing
rooms during lunch break. It's all fiction
or the sign of a personality disorder.

Eat sensibly, take your vitamins and put your
scale in the garage.

N O T E S :...

....

....

....

....

....

........12.3...............
D A T E

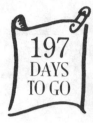

197
DAYS
TO GO

Surrender

Surrender, Dorothy! Your body is yours in name only, because a baby has moved in and taken control. And why shouldn't it assume control, since your baby knows at least as much about pregnancy as you do?

Children have a way of laying claim to a mother's body from the time they live in it until the day they steal the car keys.

N O T E S : ....
....
....
....
....
....
....

........12-4........

DATE

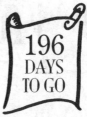

196
DAYS
TO GO

As your pregnancy progresses, it will astonish
you how much more time you spend thinking
about your baby than your husband does.
He can spend all day without finding a
single moment to obsess about baby names or
the fact that the C-section rate is at an all-time
high. So, when you have called him at work
for the tenth time today, don't be ashamed;
just think of it as "sharing."

NOTES:..
....
....
....
....
....

TOP 10 REASONS NOT TO EXERCISE

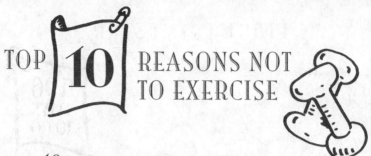

10. YOU WILL GET FATTER ANYWAY.

9. EXERCISING WILL NOT MAKE LABOR AND DELIVERY EASIER, SINCE CONTRACTIONS ARE INVOLUNTARY MOVEMENTS OF THE UTERUS, AND THE UTERUS IS A DIFFICULT MUSCLE TO TRAIN IN A GYM.

8. GRAVITY IS HARD ENOUGH ON YOUR VOLUPTUOUS BREASTS AND BUTT WHEN YOU'RE STANDING STILL, LET ALONE WHEN YOU'RE HOPPING UP AND DOWN IN A STEP AEROBICS CLASS.

7. IT'S NOT GOOD FOR THE BABY OR YOU TO GET OVERHEATED; IT STARTS TO FEEL LIKE A HARD-BOILED EGG.

6. YOUR LIGAMENTS ARE LOOSER, AND YOU CAN TWIST YOUR KNEES OR ANKLES WITH ONE WOBBLY MOVEMENT.

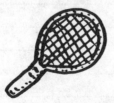

5. YOUR BODY IS WORKING FULL-TILT MANUFACTURING A HUMAN BEING; DON'T DISTRACT IT WITH LOW-IMPACT-CARDIO-FUNK-'N'-FREE-WEIGHTS CLASSES.

4. YOU MIGHT ENDANGER THE PREGNANCY. EVEN IF YOU DON'T, IF A PROBLEM APPEARS AT ANY TIME DURING GESTATION, YOU WILL ALWAYS WONDER IF IT WAS THAT SQUAT MACHINE THAT CAUSED IT.

3. OUR COMPULSION TO EXERCISE WHEN WE ARE PREGNANT IS A REFLECTION OF OUR INABILITY TO SURRENDER AND LET NATURE RUN ITS COURSE. LET THE SUBSCRIPTIONS TO YOUR FASHION MAGAZINES LAPSE TILL FURTHER NOTICE.

2. YOU ARE TOO TIRED.

1. DO YOU REALLY NEED AN EXCUSE?

FIRST TRIMESTER

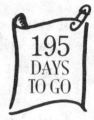

195 DAYS TO GO

You should be so proud of yourself.
Being pregnant is one of the few professions
that you can be sure you are uniquely qualified
for. No doubts about whether this job is "creative"
enough for you or allows you to "make
a difference." It's just what Mother Nature
had in mind for you, even if the pay sucks and the
hours are definitely a union violation.

NOTES: ....
....
....
....
....
....

FIRST TRIMESTER

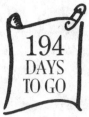

Since there is no graceful way to ask this,
I will just plunge in. Are you noticing that you are
more lubricated than you were before you were
"with child"? An increase in vaginal discharge
is normal. You might want to try
panty liners; and even if you are a panty-free
gal when you're not pregnant, you <u>must</u> wear
cotton panties when you are.

N O T E S: ....
....
....
....
....
....

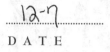

DATE

193 DAYS TO GO

Yeast infections are so common in pregnant
women you'd think they were bread-makers.
If you notice the telltale discomfort, DO NOT TRY
TO CURE IT YOURSELF BY DOUCHING.
In fact, the rule of thumb during pregnancy
is never let anything up near your cervix
except your husband or your doctor.
Call your doctor for a prescription cream
that is safe for you and the baby.

NOTES:

FIRST TRIMESTER

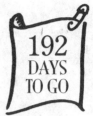

192
DAYS
TO GO

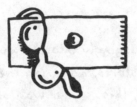

Time to clean out your drawers.
All belts and Wonderbras can be put into
storage until further notice. Never, ever, put a
belt around a body without a distinguishable
waistline or you will look like a beach umbrella
closed up around a basketball.

NOTES:...
....
....
....
....
....

FIRST TRIMESTER

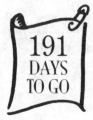

Gazing longingly into the windows of
maternity stores, admiring the fashions?
Actually, this is your way of dipping
one more toe in the Sea of Surrender.
If you fight this pregnancy stuff too hard,
you really waste a lot of energy.
Make friends with the things that
frighten you, like gussets in your pants
and panties big enough to use as pillowcases,
because they will definitely be part of your life.

NOTES:...
....
....
....
....
....

FIRST TRIMESTER

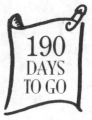

190 DAYS TO GO

Try some fresh fruit. Watermelon, nectarines, grapes and apple slices (without the peel) can taste great and stay down in your nauseous tummy. Experiment, but our Girlfriends' advice is to stick to foods that are high in water content so that you don't have to gag to get them down.

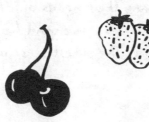

N O T E S : ....

....

....

....

....

....

FIRST TRIMESTER

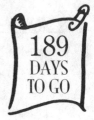

189
DAYS
TO GO

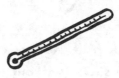

Pregnant women are hot, and I mean
that in its most literal sense. Many husbands
complain that their wives keep the house
so cold that their breath frosts and that
they must hang their heads out the car window
like the family dog. We can't help it...we are
incubators in the purest sense of the word.

N O T E S:...
....
....
....
....
....

FIRST TRIMESTER

188 DAYS TO GO

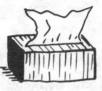

Feel like you are coming down with a cold?
You might just be coming down
with pregnancy rhinitis, also known
as chronic stuffy mommy nose.
Don't worry, it will clear up in 188 more days.

NOTES: ....
....
....
....
....
....

FIRST TRIMESTER

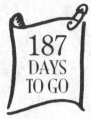

187
DAYS
TO GO

Congratulations on being a walking inspiration
of goodwill and boundless optimism
(no matter how green and crazy you feel).
Since the beginning of time, any woman who
has gotten pregnant by a man who has a job
and is not married to someone else has
been cheered as if she invented the condition.
At least the first time around.

N O T E S: ....
....
....
....
....

FIRST TRIMESTER

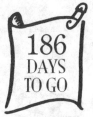

186
DAYS
TO GO

Not a big fan of milk? Worried that since you can't gag down the 24 ounces recommended by greater authorities, you're depriving your baby of the calcium it needs? First of all, if you're shortchanging anyone, it's probably you because the baby gets first dibs on your resources. Second of all, this situation can be easily handled by asking

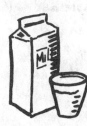

your doctor to suggest a calcium supplement. Remember, those antacids that we're so crazy about also have calcium, as do yogurt, cheese and Oreos (if dunked in milk, of course!).

N O T E S:...
....
....
....
....
....

SECOND TRIMESTER

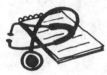

12-15
....
D A T E

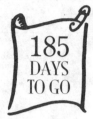

185
DAYS
TO GO

When you sat down with your gynecologist
and he miraculously became your obstetrician,
you probably received a stack of papers about the
miracle of birth. You may have read them or
thrown them in the garbage, but make sure you
locate the hospital preregistration information.
I know it seems far away, but it's one less thing
to worry about. The form is quite simple and will
make life a little less complicated when it's time
to go to the hospital. You certainly don't want to
hear them say there's no room at the inn.

N O T E S: ....
....
....
....
....
....

SECOND TRIMESTER

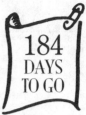

184
DAYS
TO GO

You may be wondering right about now, "If the baby is growing in my belly, why is my butt so big?"
The answer lies somewhere in Darwin's theory of evolution: When we still walked on all fours, that bubble butt provided a rumble seat for our babies. Keep this in mind when getting dressed; you should never leave the house without looking in a mirror to check out your backside.

NOTES: ....
....
....
....
....
....

SECOND TRIMESTER

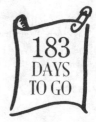

183
DAYS
TO GO

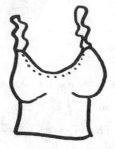

Wear something figure-revealing today.
Show off your spectacular bustline before
your tummy starts competing with it.
Remember, the day will come when the boobs
actually sit on the belly AND look
small by comparison.

NOTES: ....
....
....
....
....
....

SECOND TRIMESTER

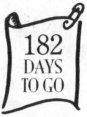

182
DAYS
TO GO

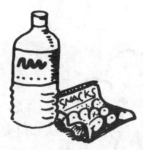

Always keep water and food in your car.
Not in case of a natural disaster, but because
pregnant means always having to say
you're hungry or thirsty.

If you haven't planned ahead and stocked up
with water, juice, trail mix or crackers, you
will be forced to pull into fast-food restaurants
and before you know it, you'll have a
Quarter-Pounder in each hand.

N O T E S: ....

....

....

....

....

....

SECOND TRIMESTER

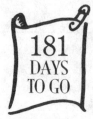

The "gas gremlins" should be invading your body any time now, if they aren't already permanent residents. Slower digestion can make you as fragrant as a barnyard animal. Just remember to say "excuse me" to anyone who has the bad taste to notice, and when it happens at night, do your husband a favor and fluff the sheets.

NOTES: ....
....
....
....
....
....

.....12 - 20.........
D A T E

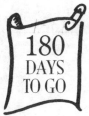

180
DAYS
TO GO

Do you wake up feeling svelte and
light in the mornings and then get fatter
and heavier as the day goes on?
Most expectant women can't wait until the
end of the day, when they can pull off
their shoes, yank off the panty hose and
ease out of the pants that have been
unzipped since lunchtime. At the top of
the pleasure heap is taking off your
bra and having a good tummy scratch.

N O T E S: ....
....
....
....
....
....

SECOND TRIMESTER

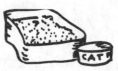

Let's talk about pets for a moment. Are you crazy about your kitty? That's all well and good, but you shouldn't be touching any dirty kitty litter because it carries critters that are dangerous to pregnant women. How about your dog that has been like a child to you all these years? Trust us when we tell you that it will rejoin the animal world once your real baby comes. One last note...if you have lizards, snakes or other reptiles, talk to several pediatricians (and a psychiatrist or two). Many doctors think that those pets carry infections that are very dangerous to babies and young children.

NOTES: ....
....
....
....
....
....

12-22

DATE

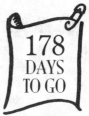

178
DAYS
TO GO

Every time you ask yourself, "Can I go one more day without having to shampoo my hair?" shout "No!" You have more hair now that you're pregnant, and it gets heavy and dull faster now. Make the extra effort because a good hair day can compensate for a bad complexion day.

NOTES:...
....
....
....
....
....

......12-23..........
DATE

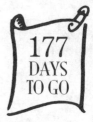

177
DAYS
TO GO

You should be getting an ultrasound soon
to see what your little darling looks like,
inside and out. You will be advised to fill
your bladder to enhance the picture, and
we're not talking a little bit filled. Just wait
until you've gulped down three eight-ounce
glasses of water and are forbidden to peepee.
Does the term "Chinese water torture" suddenly
seem more meaningful to you?

NOTES:...
....
....
....
....
....

SECOND TRIMESTER

12-24
DATE

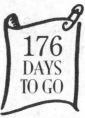
176
DAYS
TO GO

Boy? girl?

Boy or girl? Do you and your husband want
to know ahead of time? An ultrasound as early
as now could give you that information if you
want it. If you don't, make sure to tell every
single person you encounter on your way to the
ultrasound appointment, from the parking garage
attendant, to the receptionist, to the technicians,
to the doctor (who may have forgotten since
you last discussed this). People often can't conceal
their excitement when they spot a little penis on
the screen (or the absence thereof), and they
immediately start calling it "he" or "she."

NOTES:...
....
....
....
....
....

SECOND TRIMESTER

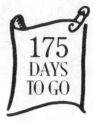

175
DAYS
TO GO

Remember: Your pregnancy is not your
mother's pregnancy. She probably smoked and
drank and kept her coffee habit when she
was pregnant with you, she was asleep when
you were born and she recuperated in the
hospital for a week or two afterward. So, if
she starts telling you that you're neurotic
about microwaves and NutraSweet, or that
you're getting way too fat, ignore her.

N O T E S : ....
....
....
....
....
....

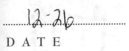

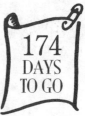

174
DAYS
TO GO

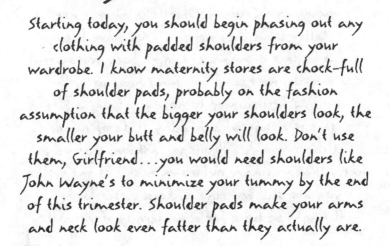

Starting today, you should begin phasing out any clothing with padded shoulders from your wardrobe. I know maternity stores are chock-full of shoulder pads, probably on the fashion assumption that the bigger your shoulders look, the smaller your butt and belly will look. Don't use them, Girlfriend...you would need shoulders like John Wayne's to minimize your tummy by the end of this trimester. Shoulder pads make your arms and neck look even fatter than they actually are.

NOTES:...
....
....
....
....

SECOND TRIMESTER

173
DAYS
TO GO

To paraphrase a common automotive
warning, "Caution: Objects in mirror are
fatter than they appear." You have been
living in this growing, changing body for several
months now, and you may have actually
become accustomed to how you look. While
this is a sign of a healthy state of mind,
it can prove disastrous in fashion. It is very
likely that you have outgrown many of the clothes
you are still wearing. Take a closer look...
it might be time for a maternity store visit.

NOTES:

SECOND TRIMESTER

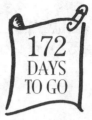

172
DAYS
TO GO

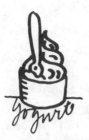

Doesn't food taste fabulous these days?
You wolf down with enthusiasm even "good for
you" stuff like salads. You know how we
Girlfriends feel about watching our weight during
pregnancy—deeply offended—so we are nothing but
happy for you and your local frozen yogurt parlor.

One word of caution, however: Many men get
cranky if you eat the food off their plates after
you have hoovered your own. No matter how good
those french fries look sitting before him,
keep your hands off.

N O T E S: ....
....
....
....
....
....

SECOND TRIMESTER

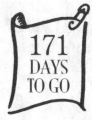

How's your skin doing? If you have been battling
pimples, you might be finding that your skin is
clearer. On the other hand, you may start to notice
patches of darker skin across your nose and
cheeks. This is called <u>chloasma</u>, but it is more
sinisterly known as the "mask of pregnancy"
(as if it provided any kind of disguise
whatsoever!). This is just another pregnancy thing,
and there isn't much you can do about it, except
wear sunblock even when the only light you
see comes from inside the refrigerator.

NOTES: ....
....
....
....
....

SECOND TRIMESTER

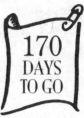

170
DAYS
TO GO

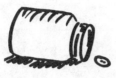

Are you taking iron supplements along with or
in your prenatal vitamins? If you are, this
iron might be contributing to the constipation
that plagues most pregnant women. It is also
to blame for the unfamiliarly dark poops you
may have noticed. I used to think it looked
like tire rubber, myself.

Ask your doctor if you can take a break
from iron for a while, or if a stool softener
could be your salvation.

NOTES:...
....
....
....
....
....

SECOND TRIMESTER

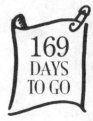

Amniocentesis (am-nee-oh-cen-TEE-sis) is
traditionally performed around the sixteenth
week of pregnancy in women who are over age
thirty-five or who have a history of genetic
problems. It can be done in your doctor's office
or at a lab that specializes in such procedures.
It is done by drawing amniotic fluid out
through a very long needle in your belly.

Does this hurt? Surprisingly, no. Is it creepy?
Yes, so bring someone into the room with
you to distract you with droll conversation
and discuss the images on the ultrasound monitor
with you..."Is that a leg or a penis?"

N O T E S: ....
....
....
....
....
....

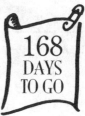

168
DAYS
TO GO

Stay in bed the day of and the day after your amnio. Sure, you probably feel fine, just exhausted by the small nervous breakdown you had before the procedure, but you must rest anyway. You have just sprung a small leak, and only a person who thinks pregnancy is something to be overcome, rather than accepted, would even consider leaping up to go back to the office or stock up on a few things from Costco.

Besides, once the baby is born, you will never be allowed to lie in bed to recuperate from anything short of open-heart surgery.

N O T E S:..
....
....
....
....
....

SECOND TRIMESTER

It usually takes ten days to two weeks to get the results of your amniocentesis...easily the longest two weeks of your existence. There isn't really much we can suggest to help you endure this trial; just stay as busy as you can, and remember how overwhelmingly in your favor the odds of perfection really are.

Don't fool yourself into thinking that the good results from your amnio will leave you worry-free for the rest of your pregnancy. Your fertile mind will move right on to unsightly birthmarks, hearing difficulties, even the big nose you once had. Remember, nothing can live up to your vivid imagination.

N O T E S : ....

....

....

....

....

....

SECOND TRIMESTER

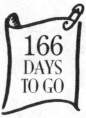

166
DAYS
TO GO

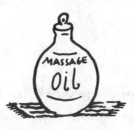

MASSAGE
OIL

Here's the news: The only way to prevent stretch
marks is to pick your mother carefully.
You see, a propensity toward those maligned
marks is genetic. You can massage gallons
of potions, lotions and health food store oils into
your skin, and you will still get stretch marks if
that's what nature had in mind for you.

The general rule is: Oil massages don't prevent
stretch marks, they create pregnancies.

N O T E S:...
....
....
....
....
....

SECOND TRIMESTER

This time of pregnancy often brings such a
sense of well-being and vigor that you might feel
even more terrific than you do when you're not
pregnant. Lots of Girlfriends report that their
immunity to colds and flus is stronger, their energy
is boundless and they feel sexy and aroused.
Of course, this could be an exaggerated response
to the relief they feel at not being sick and tired
like they were in the first trimester. Either
way, if you are feeling exceptionally well,
live it up because you may not feel this great
again till your next pregnancy.

N O T E S : ....
....
....
....
....
....

SECOND TRIMESTER

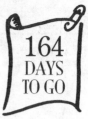

164
DAYS
TO GO

Now that you are feeling better, it's time to
consider your pregnancy exercise routine.
Our suggestion is elegant in its simplicity and ease:
Give up all exercise classes, free weights,
climbers and thigh-masters. Swim if you must,
or take a walk now and then, but don't buy into
that brainwashing that says exercising will help
prepare you for labor and delivery, unless
Nautilus has invented a uterus machine
since my last visit to the gym.

N O T E S: ....
....
....
....
....
....

SECOND TRIMESTER

163
DAYS
TO GO

By virtue of being a non-female, your
husband will have absolutely no idea what
it feels like to be in your shoes. He will not
truly know your anxiety, your ambivalence,
your insecurities or your near-toxic hormonal
state. That's enough right there to qualify him
for the title of World's Most Annoying Man.
All we can offer is the assurance that
he's no worse than most, and he will look
a lot better with his baby in his arms.

N O T E S: ....
....
....
....
....
....

SECOND TRIMESTER

162
DAYS
TO GO

Sex is beginning to look a lot more interesting, isn't it? First of all, you are probably coming off a long, dry spell, what with all that nausea, fatigue and atomic titties. Second, your pregnancy hormones are settling into a nice little aphrodisiac cocktail. And it can't hurt that your "privates" are chronically engorged with blood, a state they used to be able to achieve only through foreplay. Your body is your sex toy and your husband your slave. Have fun while it lasts!

N O T E S: ....
....
....
....
....
....

SECOND TRIMESTER

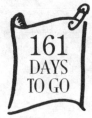

161
DAYS
TO GO

The Girlfriends recommend the top position
for pregnant sex. This allows you to present your
breasts in a tantalizing way and keep your lumpy
rear end where it belongs...out of sight.

Best of all, this position gives you control over
how deep the penetration goes...and really,
control is everything, isn't it?

N O T E S: ....

....

....

....

....

....

SECOND TRIMESTER

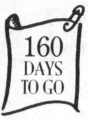

160
DAYS
TO GO

Lots of Girlfriends have very sexy dreams
during this part of pregnancy. Not just sexy,
like, say, a Barbara Cartland novel.
No, we're talking Pussycat Theater stuff, all in
your own little imagination.

When you awaken after one of these doozies, it
won't be to make yet another trip to the bathroom,
but to attack your unsuspecting husband
for a reenactment.

N O T E S:...
....
....
....
....
....

SECOND TRIMESTER

For Girlfriends experiencing a sexual renaissance, the general rules of thumb are:

1. Quick to arouse (in fact, some say in constant state of arousal).

2. Slower to climax.

3. And when you do climax, it is like a 9.0 on the Richter scale, with several aftershocks, courtesy of Mother (of course) Nature.

NOTES: ....
....
....
....
....
....

SECOND TRIMESTER

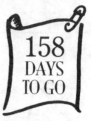

158
DAYS
TO GO

There isn't much in the way of sexy
maternity lingerie, but you are probably still
small enough to wear larger sizes of real people's
lingerie. The idea is to emphasize the
breasts and conceal the hips and butt.
Think empire waists or a bra and panties
peeking out of a robe or kimono.
By the time the robe comes off, odds are good
that the lights will be off or the covers can
be artfully arranged over your fanny.

NOTES: ....
....
....
....
....
....

SECOND TRIMESTER

157
DAYS
TO GO

Sex, if you're indeed having sex,
gets more physically challenging in your
fifth and sixth months of pregnancy. Even if your
belly does not protrude enough to create a
barricade between you and your mate, it is
probably heavy enough to make you feel like
fainting when you lie flat on your back.

For heaven's sake, don't let this stop you!
Try some position other than missionary.
One Girlfriends' favorite is called "spoons," and
it involves the two of you lying on your sides,
facing in the same direction, with your fella
behind you. Any "rear" approach will work,
but many women think that "doggy style" hurts
because of that deeper penetration.

NOTES: ....
....
....
....
....
....

SECOND TRIMESTER

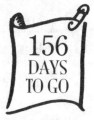

156
DAYS
TO GO

If you are, indeed, feeling more like your old
self, don't share that information with your
husband. He will feel so relieved that his "real"
wife has come back that he will be less concerned
about you and begin to take you for granted.
Men can forget they are pregnant for hours on
end, and it is our job to keep that from happening.
Don't ever let him labor under the delusion
that gestating is part-time work.

NOTES:
....
....
....
....
....
....

SECOND TRIMESTER

155
DAYS
TO GO

It is not considered bad form to use your
pregnancy as an excuse or special circumstance,
but if you don't look undeniably pregnant yet,
you must speak up and state your needs.
You might consider trying it out on public
transportation (unless, of course, you live in
New York), on a police officer who has
stopped you for speeding ("My blood sugar
was dropping and I needed to hurry to the
nearest fast-food restaurant!") or in a snooty
boutique that refuses to share its bathroom.
It goes without saying that you should use it on
your husband any time you want since he won't
fall for it for any pregnancy after this one.

N O T E S:..
....
....
....
....
....

SECOND TRIMESTER

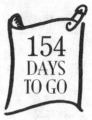

154
DAYS
TO GO

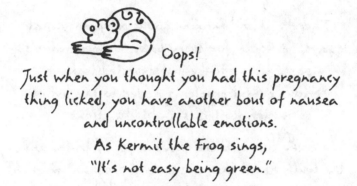

Oops!
Just when you thought you had this pregnancy
thing licked, you have another bout of nausea
and uncontrollable emotions.
As Kermit the Frog sings,
"It's not easy being green."

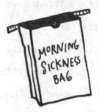

MORNING
SICKNESS
BAG

N O T E S:..
....
....
....
....
....

SECOND TRIMESTER

153
DAYS
TO GO

There's an old maxim about pregnancy that
says, "A tooth for every baby." In generations
past, moms-to-be just expected to have
serious dental problems added to the list of
maternity trials and tribulations.

In every cliché, there is a nugget of truth, and
the truth about this one is that pregnant women
must pay particular attention to their teeth, and
perhaps more specifically, their gums. You may
notice your gums bleed easily when you brush
them. This can lead to infection and decay if
you don't consult your dentist at least twice
during pregnancy and follow her orders.

N O T E S: ....

....

....

....

....

....

SECOND TRIMESTER

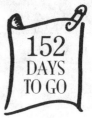

152
DAYS
TO GO

Take a good look at your legs in a three-way mirror before leaving the house in bike shorts or a miniskirt. Some long-limbed pregnant Girlfriends can show off their legs all summer long, but those of us who are described in fashion magazines as "pear-shaped" tend to get enough cellulite to make our thighs look like relief maps of Switzerland.

NOTES:..
....
....
....
....
....

SECOND TRIMESTER

151 DAYS TO GO

This is generally about the time when people start talking to you about a baby shower, unless you are Jewish, in which case they start planning for the bris. Showers are great and are to be encouraged since no one can really afford all the baby paraphernalia you think you'll need.

Our advice is: Don't accept too quickly offers to throw your shower. If you are lucky enough to have more than one party-loving friend, you should wait and weigh all offers until about the sixth month and have them throw you a shower together.

NOTES:..
....
....
....
....
....

SECOND TRIMESTER

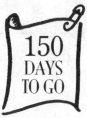

150
DAYS
TO GO

This pregnancy business isn't half bad, is it?
In fact, you might begin to wonder at this point
what all those other pregnant women have
been moaning and complaining about.
You can carry this off...no problem.
Lots of energy, not too fat. Secure in
your ability to become a mother, you feel like
a million bucks, right? Hey, it's us you're
talking to, Girlfriend, get real!

N O T E S:...
....
....
....
....
....

SECOND TRIMESTER

149
DAYS
TO GO

Even though the common prohibition against pregnant women stewing in hot tubs and Jacuzzis makes good sense, your own friendly home bathtub can be your best friend right up until your water breaks or you lose your mucous plug.

The critical difference between your bathroom tub and the health club Jacuzzi, leaving out for the moment our morbid fear of the bacteria of strangers, is that the Jacuzzi does not cool off and your tub does. It's that exposure to unrelenting heat that can dangerously raise your core body temperature.

N O T E S: ....
....
....
....
....
....

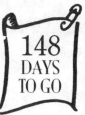

148
DAYS
TO GO

Until they know and adore them personally, most men tend to think of babies as shortcuts to the poorhouse. They know how much food kids eat (especially teenagers), they assume a new home is looming in their future, and anyone who has read _Time_ magazine knows that college in eighteen years will cost more than that looming new home. All this worrying is good; it distracts them and makes the pregnancy pass more quickly.

N O T E S: ....
....
....
....
....
....

1-22

D A T E

147
DAYS
TO GO

Pregnancy is as good a time as any to settle
your issues with your own mother. You may
have your mother's chin or her laugh or her
butt, but you are not your mother.
Here's your chance to appraise your own
childhood and pick and choose the parts you
want to share with your kids and the
parts you want to spare them.

N O T E S: ....

....

....

....

....

....

SECOND TRIMESTER

146
DAYS
TO GO

Lots of pregnant women have a secret fear that they will be a bad mother. Either their own mother was so extraordinarily loving, patient and selfless that they know they could never, in a million years, be as good as she was...or their mother was such a selfish, neglectful and undemonstrative person that they are terrified they may be genetically predisposed to act just like her. Take heart, your baby will think you're perfect for at least ten or eleven years.

N O T E S: ....

....

....

....

....

....

SECOND TRIMESTER

145
DAYS
TO GO

There is no predicting what your
pregnancy will be like, just as there
is no deep instinctual knowledge about
giving birth or nursing a baby.
Just make it up as you go along;
everybody else does.

NOTES: ....
....
....
....
....
....

SECOND TRIMESTER

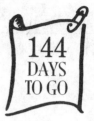

144
DAYS
TO GO

Some women take this pregnancy
purity business a tad too far.
Sure, we are unanimous in the righteousness
of giving up smoking and drug use and
we are fairly unanimous about not drinking.
We start splitting ranks over microwaved food,
airport security, coffee and sugar.
And we have had it up to here with
women who freak out about chemicals
in crib mattresses and the use of
Novocain for dental work. The idea is to
be protective, not paranoid.

NOTES:...

....

....

....

....

....

SECOND TRIMESTER

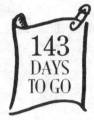

143
DAYS
TO GO

Lots of women in your shoes (which, by the way, must be feeling a bit tight) are frustrated that they don't look pregnant enough to look...well, pregnant. Your friends who have children already will smile wickedly and say "Just wait...". But you can't believe that you are already five months pregnant and you don't look ripe with child.

First of all, let me remind you that pregnancy is a ten-month affair, so you still have plenty of time for expansion. I promise you that you will not reach the end of the pregnancy feeling gypped that you didn't get big enough.

NOTES:...
....
....
....
....
....

SECOND TRIMESTER

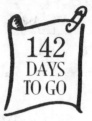

142
DAYS
TO GO

Can you feel the baby moving yet? Maybe
you think you have been feeling it for a couple of
weeks, but have just now become certain that
it's the baby and not gas. Either way, feeling the
presence of your child is out of this world.
The Girlfriends agree that, of all the experiences
of pregnancy, feeling the baby move is the one
we miss the most (or, in some cases, the only
thing we miss). It's like having a wonderful
secret; you feel kind of smug, like when you're
the only one at a party who knows that
you aren't wearing underwear.

N O T E S: ....
....
....
....
....
....

SECOND TRIMESTER

141
DAYS
TO GO

Kerri

Dawn

Don

Rarely are husbands and wives unanimous
about anything from whether to share the
Caesar salad for two in a restaurant to
what show to watch on television. Why on earth
would you expect to agree on the baby's name?
Actually, the ideal time to lobby for _your_
favorite name is during labor, when your
husband is terrified and will do
anything to comfort you.

Jack

Alvin

NOTES:

SECOND TRIMESTER

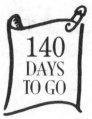

140
DAYS
TO GO

Lucy

Paul

Mae

We moms obsess over baby names.
So why is it your husband seems so
unconcerned with this baby-naming business?
What does he think...
that they hand out names at the hospital?

James

Eloise

N O T E S:..
....
....
....
....
....

SECOND TRIMESTER

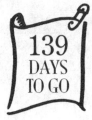

139
DAYS
TO GO

If you are exceptions to the rule and you and
your husband have settled on a name for the baby,
don't tell it to anyone, no matter how they beg!
People feel completely free to challenge your
selection at any time before the moniker is
typed onto the birth certificate. Your beloved
name will inevitably be the same as that of the
little girl in your brother-in-law's second-grade
class who picked her nose and ate it.

After the baby and its name have bonded, no one
will dare say anything unflattering about your
choice, no matter how bad it is.

N O T E S : ....

....

....

....

....

....

SECOND TRIMESTER

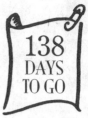

138 DAYS TO GO

Some books, especially those written by
people who have never been pregnant, describe
the sensation of the baby moving within you
as gas. This is not very accurate. It feels like there
is a feather or a cotton ball stroking or tapping
you on the inside. It can also be a lurching
sensation, like when you are startled.
Think roller coaster on flat land.

NOTES: ....
....
....
....
....
....

SECOND TRIMESTER

137
DAYS
TO GO

"Braxton Hicks Contractions" are contractions of the uterus during pregnancy that <u>do not</u> open up your cervix. Later, you may be told you are having "false labor" when your abdomen gets hard enough to bounce nickels off it, but there is nothing false about them. They are, in fact, good preparation for labor. The good news is that they don't really hurt, but they really can grab your attention.

NOTES: ....

....

....

....

....

SECOND TRIMESTER

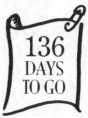

136
DAYS
TO GO

Be brave. It is time for your first
visit to a maternity store as a real
customer. I know, your belly
doesn't stick <u>that</u> far out yet, but
at the rate you're growing, you won't
realize you're a candidate for elastic
waist pants with a panel until you are
half-dressed and crying in your closet because
you can't find anything that fits.

NOTES: ....
....
....
....
....
....

SECOND TRIMESTER

135
DAYS
TO GO

Lots of otherwise intelligent people maintain
that you can make your baby smarter and more
closely bonded with you if you and your husband
speak to it in your tummy. Our guess is that
babies' grasp of English is still minimal, so they
don't really know which of our many conversations
throughout the day are directed at them. That
means you are probably meeting your New Age
maternal obligations simply by letting the little
fetus eavesdrop on your telephone conversations.

One thing does seem certain: Your newborn
will recognize your voice and quiet down to hear it,
even in the delivery room.

N O T E S : ....
....
....
....
....
....

SECOND TRIMESTER

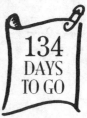

134
DAYS
TO GO

Some women notice an increase in their
saliva production, of all unnecessary functions,
when they are pregnant.
Carry a supply of hard candy to keep up
the sucking action, and Kleenex to catch any
spillover. Otherwise, you will end up
talking like Tweety's friend, Sylvester:
"Ssssufferin' ssssuccotash!"

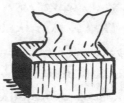

NOTES:...
....
....
....
....
....

..........2-5..........
DATE

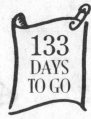

133 DAYS TO GO

6 WEEK LEAVE Are you a little nervous about discussing maternity leave with your boss? Or are you even more nervous because you don't really know if you plan to go back to work at all after the baby is born? Trust our combined Girlfriends' experience when we say that the way the system works, you pretty much have to say you are returning to work immediately after your maternity leave, no matter what your real plans are. That means that you will receive your legislated paid six weeks, but anything other than that is usually stated in your employer's handbook or negotiated.

NOTES:..
....
....
....
....
....

SECOND TRIMESTER

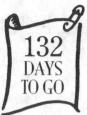

132
DAYS
TO GO

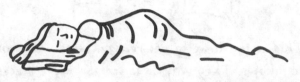

It is now time to learn to sleep on your side,
your left side in particular. You already probably
feel weird sleeping on your tummy for fear of
squishing anybody, but your back is becoming
inappropriate now, too. Even before you can feel
the effects, the baby is getting heavy enough to put
a kink in the main artery that runs from your
heart down into your legs, much like when a car
tire runs over the garden hose. It will take you a
while to adapt to this single sleep option, but
fatigue always overcomes a little discomfort.

N O T E S: ....
....
....
....
....
....

SECOND TRIMESTER

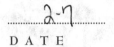
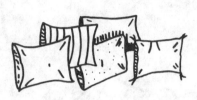

131
DAYS
TO GO

This is the time to get reacquainted with your bed pillows. They will no longer be mere pieces of furniture, but rather dear and valued friends. And, as we all know, you can never have too many friends. Most Girlfriends report being intimate with up to five pillows a night.

Here is how to arrange your little slumber group: two soft pillows under your head (helps fight heartburn and a stuffy nose), one between your knees to support your loose hips and one against your tummy. There may not be much room left for your husband, but, hey, pregnancy is hard on all of us.

N O T E S : ....

....

....

....

....

....

SECOND TRIMESTER

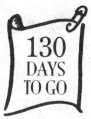

130
DAYS
TO GO

Go ahead and buy maternity panty hose and
leggings. I know you think you can still squeeze
into your old ones, but if you bend over or sneeze,
you will find the waistband rolled up tight just
above your pubic hair.
Get the ones designed for your belly.

NOTES:...
....
....
....
....
....

SECOND TRIMESTER

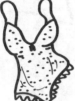

You deserve to swim, even if you don't look like a <u>Sports Illustrated</u> swimsuit model anymore. That's why you should invest in a maternity swimsuit. By the end of this trimester, even a larger size of your traditional non-maternity suit will not be up to the job. Your belly needs more fabric than regular suits provide, plus your glorious breasts will thank you for the extra support a maternity suit provides.

<u>Girlfriends' Note</u>: Use a hand mirror to check your pubic area; otherwise, you may be overdue for a wax or shave and not know it because your belly has hidden it.

N O T E S: ....

....

....

....

....

....

SECOND TRIMESTER

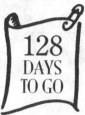

128
DAYS
TO GO

Remember your first trimester, when you
began to see veins where you'd never seen
them before, like your breasts? Well, Girlfriend,
by this time, you might also have noticed
them on your legs. Yes, I am doing my best to
ease you into the topic of varicose veins. Quick,
sit down before we go on. Yes, they look
pretty ghastly, and they can hurt, but I
promise things will vastly improve after the
baby is born. In the meantime, invest in several
pairs of maternity support hose and sit with
your feet up at every possible opportunity.

NOTES:..
....
....
....
....
....

SECOND TRIMESTER

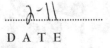

127 DAYS TO GO

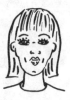

The only exercises that you must commit to are Kegels. They are intended to strengthen the muscles in your pelvic floor, which is somewhere around your vagina, cervix and bladder. This is the front line of defense against incontinence and a loosey-goosey vagina after delivery.

You can identify these muscles by stopping the flow of urine when you're on the toilet. The mental image should be of an elevator moving up from your labia to behind your navel. You'll know you're doing these exercises right if they make you feel a little anxious by the time the muscles get to the top floor.

N O T E S: ....
....
....
....
....
....

SECOND TRIMESTER

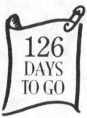

126 DAYS TO GO

You know the balloon animals that clowns make at birthday parties? Take a look at your hands and feet. Notice any resemblance? That is what is known as water retention. Many pregnant women end up having to remove their wedding rings by the third trimester because they are too tight. Consider this just another good reason to sit with your feet up and your hands idle.

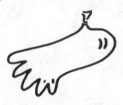

N O T E S: ....
....
....
....
....
....

SECOND TRIMESTER

125
DAYS
TO GO

Stretch marks might be artfully decorating
your breasts, belly and butt, and you feel like
killing the great artist on high. While these
marks won't go away, they will improve
tremendously in the year after the baby is born,
especially if you keep them out of the sun.
Just as heroes in the military earn stripes,
so do the heroes of maternity, and they
should be worn with at least as much pride.

NOTES: ....
....
....
....
....
....

TOP 10 PREGNANCY FASHION VIOLATIONS

10. JUMPSUITS (THINK BOZO).

9. ANYTHING WITH LARGE BUTTONS IN CONTRASTING COLORS, SAILOR COLLARS OR BIG LOOPY BOWS.

8. DRESSES OR BLOUSES BELTED.

7. CAP SLEEVES.

6. SHOULDER PADS.

5. BIRKENSTOCKS.

4. JACKETS THAT ARE NOT LONG ENOUGH TO COVER YOUR THIGHS.

3. PANTY HOSE IN ANY COLOR OTHER THAN BLACK.

2. STIRRUPS THAT SHOW ABOVE THE SHOE.

1. T-SHIRTS WITH WITTY SAYINGS LIKE "BABY ON BOARD" OR "I'M NOT FAT, I'M PREGNANT!"

SECOND TRIMESTER

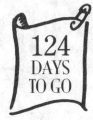

124
DAYS
TO GO

The Girlfriends support legislation
requiring all visibly pregnant women to
wear opaque stockings, preferably black, when
their legs are visible. Trust us in this, unless
you are certain that you have no protruding
veins, a flawless, even color and no extra
padding at the knees and thighs.

N O T E S: ....
....
....
....
....
....

SECOND TRIMESTER

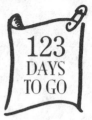

123
DAYS
TO GO

Let's talk about pants with stirrups.
They are ubiquitous in maternity fashion,
and with good reason, because they give your
legs a longer, less bumpy appearance. But there
is a hard and fast rule. Never, ever, wear shoes
that show the stirrup. Wear boots, or even big
gym socks, but don't have that little pudgy part of
your pregnant foot on display. If you can't wear
boots, at least promise us that you will wear
opaque panty hose that match the pants.

NOTES:

SECOND TRIMESTER

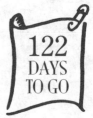

122 DAYS TO GO

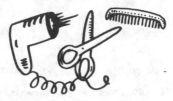

Right about now, you may be thinking about getting a new hairdo. You know, something shorter, bouncier, easier to care for when the baby comes. STOP RIGHT THERE, GIRLFRIEND! What you're looking for can't be found in any beauty parlor. No hairdresser on this planet can give you a "do" that makes you look thin, energetic and well-rested at this point, so wait until the baby comes and your judgment is more reliable.

NOTES:..
....
....
....
....
....

SECOND TRIMESTER

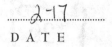
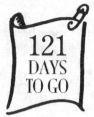

121
DAYS
TO GO

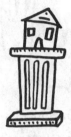

Pregnancy and the need to remodel or redecorate go hand in hand. Something in the progesterone makes women want to rip up their carpeting, install a walk-in shower or repaint the entire house. Whatever the project, it is guaranteed to take nearly forty weeks to accomplish, just so that it will be a dead heat which is finished first— the baby or the new den.

N O T E S: ....
....
....
....
....
....

SECOND TRIMESTER

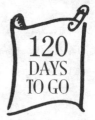

120
DAYS
TO GO

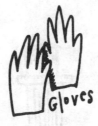

Gloves

Itchy skin is the pregnant woman's crucible.
With all that stretching your skin's
enduring, it's a wonder it doesn't complain
even more emphatically. Lotions will help,
and your doctor may suggest one with an
antihistamine in it. If you are clawing yourself,
here is a Girlfriends' tip:
Put on cotton gloves before you settle in for a nice
scratch...you will be less apt to draw blood.

N O T E S : ....
....
....
....
....
....

119
DAYS
TO GO

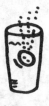

Here is today's addition to your pregnancy vocabulary: <u>acid reflux</u>, also known as "heartburn." This nasty condition occurs when the natural closure that keeps your stomach acids down in your stomach instead of up near your throat surrenders to the pressure of your rising uterus.

If your doctor is the least bit compassionate, you will be encouraged to take antacids for relief. These chalky little morsels really do help, and you should keep them everywhere, from your purse to your desk drawer to your glove compartment, and especially your bedside table.

N O T E S : ....
....
....
....
....
....

SECOND TRIMESTER

118
DAYS
TO GO

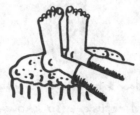

When in doubt, sit down, put your feet up
and turn so that you are lying on your hip
rather than your tush. This posture, casual
though it may look, is serious medicine.

First, it gives your swaybacked spine a break.
Second, it helps in the battle against water-
retaining ankles and takes a load off your back.
Third, if no one has noticed you sitting there yet,
you could sneak in a little nap.

NOTES:
....
....
....
....
....

SECOND TRIMESTER

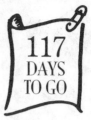

117
DAYS
TO GO

The Girlfriends' advice for today is: "Let your
mothers into your pregnancy." If you are fortunate
enough to have a mother and/or mother-in-law
on this earth, no matter how judgmental and
annoying, try getting to know her on this new level.
As you become a mother, we guarantee you
will gain a new tolerance and insight into why
your own mother is such a nut, because you
will turn into one, too. Not only will your mothers
love your angel with fierce devotion...
they may even baby-sit if begged.

N O T E S:...
....
....
....
....
....

SECOND TRIMESTER

If you have taken the Girlfriends' advice and asked for your mother's help after the baby is born, have her come a week or two <u>after</u> the baby is born, when your adrenaline is wearing off and the baby is waking up. You and your little family deserve a few days to discover each other and set up your life without parental intrusion. Besides, babies don't even <u>begin</u> to act colicky until they are three weeks old.

NOTES: ....
....
....
....
....
....

SECOND TRIMESTER

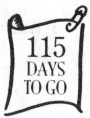

115
DAYS
TO GO

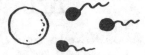

Thinking back on it now, do you think you know the precise moment when you conceived? Lots of otherwise rational women insist they felt something shift in the universe the instant the sperm crashed into the egg. Personally, I was so out of tune with the life cycle that I thought I was experiencing early menopause when I became pregnant with my daughter, but I don't doubt for a moment the veracity of my more cosmically conscious Girlfriends.

NOTES: ....
....
....
....
....

SECOND TRIMESTER

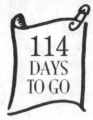

114
DAYS
TO GO

Now is a good time to figure out your living
accommodations for when you turn into a
family. Given your financial situation, can you
afford to move? Can you afford not to?
Do you need to do some work around the house?
Extra space for live-in help? Don't put these
things off and don't even think about leaving
this until after the baby comes, imagining you'll
have so much free time—because you won't.

N O T E S: ....
....
....
....
....
....

SECOND TRIMESTER

Just because your husband refuses to read
the pregnancy books you leave on his side of the
bed, and shows little enthusiasm for accompanying
you every month to the obstetrician, doesn't mean
he will be an indifferent father. Many people,
men in particular, don't romanticize the biology
of pregnancy. Don't worry, he'll come around
when the baby does.

NOTES:...
....
....
....
....
....

SECOND TRIMESTER

Trust your Girlfriends when we tell you that,
even if he denies it on a stack of Bibles,
your husband secretly thinks pregnancy has
made you irrational, emotional and
unpredictable...three things he least likes in a
person, especially a wife. Don't take it
personally...he's just terrified.

N O T E S: ....
....
....
....
....
....

SECOND TRIMESTER

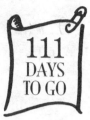

111
DAYS
TO GO

Spending way too much time reading about pregnancy so you can imagine every possible horrendous disease that could afflict your baby? Once you've worked your way through <u>eczema</u> and <u>heat rash</u>, you still have <u>roseola</u> and <u>scarlet fever</u> waiting patiently for you. As my grandmother always said, "You don't have to buy trouble, they're giving it away for free." Relax and count your blessings.

P.S. Let us save you the trouble of looking up the diseases we just mentioned, you poor, frantic thing. A DOCTOR CAN CURE ALL OF THEM!

N O T E S: ....
....
....
....
....
....

SECOND TRIMESTER

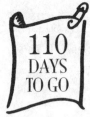

110
DAYS
TO GO

It's...Kegel Time! You might be so distracted
and forgetful at this point in your life that
you have totally neglected your pelvic floor,
but that's what Girlfriends are for. We are here
to remind you that if you want to have great
orgasms, satisfy your husband sexually
and refrain from tinkling every time you
sneeze, the key to that kingdom is the Kegel.
Try holding to a count of fifteen.

NOTES: ....
....
....
....
....
....

SECOND TRIMESTER

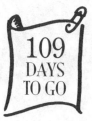

109
DAYS
TO GO

Surrender

Pregnancy is a total body experience. You must
be shocked on a daily basis about how much
control that little tyrant in your tummy has over
the rest of you. Your emotions, your complexion,
your sex drive and your hair growth are all
affected by your baby. This is when you must
learn to surrender and realize that this child
has you in its spell until the day you die.

NOTES:..
....
....
....
....
....

SECOND TRIMESTER

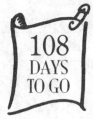

108 DAYS TO GO

Now that you are starting to show, people (even total strangers...even men!) will feel compelled to pat your belly. If you don't mind, good, because you have several more months of it coming. If you do mind, immediately cross your arms over your tummy and explain that pregnancy has made you incredibly ticklish and you'll wet your pants if touched.

NOTES: ....
....
....
....
....
....

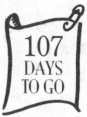

107
DAYS
TO GO

One of the more jolting pregnancy experiences is leg cramps or charley horses in your calves. One minute you are in bed, and <u>zap</u>...the back of your lower leg feels as though it's been grabbed by a giant lobster with hot claws.

Slowly stand up and put your hands against the wall to support yourself, then step backward as far as you can stretch while keeping your heels on the floor, at an angle to the wall. Tread from one foot to the other till the mutinous muscles have relaxed, then climb back into bed, being careful not to point your toes. Some people say more calcium in your diet will help...but, who knows?

NOTES:...
....
....
....
....
....

SECOND TRIMESTER

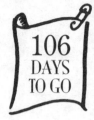

During this fragile time in your life,
try to avoid all news stories or made-for-TV
movies that portray bad things happening to
children. Pregnant women have been known
to take to their beds after hearing
Sally Struthers' pleas. We all know the world
is not a perfect place, but mommies-to-be
really need to focus inward on a world
where they have some influence.

N O T E S: ....
....
....
....
....
....

SECOND TRIMESTER

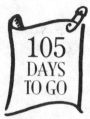

105
DAYS
TO GO

Snap out of it!
See, it really is a safe bet for me to assume
you were in one of your trancelike states.
You know what I'm talking about…
that place where everything and everyone
revolves around your pregnancy. It's like
being the star of your own movie,
as well as everyone else's.

NOTES:

SECOND TRIMESTER

DATE 3-6

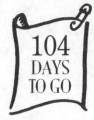

104 DAYS TO GO

Don't buy anything for your baby yet.
First of all, it's considered bad luck.
Second, you don't need anything now.
Third, even if you do need something soon,
you have no idea which brand is best and
which stores have the lowest prices.

Relax. You can start accumulating stuff next
month. Remember, the earlier you start spending
money, the more in debt you will get because no
one ever wakes up in her seventh month and
announces, "That's it! No more shopping for the
baby! I have every single thing I need!"

NOTES: ....
....
....
....
....
....

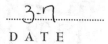

..........3-7..........

D A T E

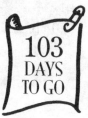

103
DAYS
TO GO

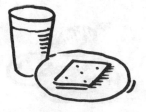

Attention all you Girlfriends who can't watch
a butt-master infomercial without feeling like you
should be exercising! Growing an entire human
being in your belly is plenty of exertion for one
woman. Besides, you're <u>supposed</u> to get fatter!
So give yourself a break and have
some milk and cookies.

N O T E S: ....
....
....
....
....
....

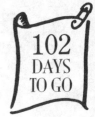

102
DAYS
TO GO

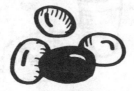

If your yearning for sweets is a
little out of hand, try a jelly bean.
Four of them (enough to get through a sugar
crisis) are only about fifteen calories and no fat.
Better still, they mask the bad taste in your
mouth when your lazy esophagus has been
leaking your lunch for the last hour.
Sure, fruit is even better, but you don't
need me to tell you that.

N O T E S: ....

....

....

....

....

....

3-9

DATE

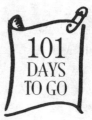

101 DAYS TO GO

You're right...it was your husband
who did this to you,
and he owes you endless
hours of attention and pampering!

N O T E S: ....

....

....

....

....

....

SECOND TRIMESTER

100
DAYS
TO GO

Repeat this over and over until you believe it:
"My due date means nothing.
My due date means nothing."

Remember, the magical date the doctor divines on
that adorable little cardboard wheel is just an
estimation, not a booking like a haircut or a plane
flight. You cannot plan your days around it like
you would around elective surgery. Get used to the
baby having this kind of influence over you...
it will continue for the rest of your life.

N O T E S: ....
....
....
....
....
....

SECOND TRIMESTER

99
DAYS
TO GO

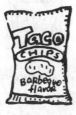

The universe is not just not fair.
If you accept that, you will be better able
to accept that it is, indeed, possible for PMS
to last forty weeks. Don't ask, "Why me?"
You don't want to go there...
just tear open another bag of
taco-flavored chips and forget about it.

NOTES:

SECOND TRIMESTER

98
DAYS
TO GO

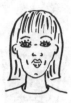

Whenever you are driving and you come
to a red light, do a Kegel and try to hold
it until the light turns green. This may
seem impossible at first, especially at busy
intersections, but it's a goal. Remember,
we're fighting giggle-peeing here, not to
mention trying to preserve your
future sex life.

N O T E S : ....
....
....
....
....
....

3-13
....
D A T E

97
DAYS
TO GO

Have you had a moment of questionable
judgment when you actually considered having a
home birth? Put that thought right out of
your head, especially if this is your first child.
Delivery is grisly business. Why would you want
to ruin your mattress and beautiful sheets?
Don't worry, you'll be home soon enough.

N O T E S : ....
....
....
....
....
....

SECOND TRIMESTER

96
DAYS
TO GO

Appetites are ferocious in pregnant women.
You're never "just a little hungry,"
and you never "sort of" have to go to the
bathroom. This is the "I want it and
I want it now" phase of maternity.

NOTES: ....

....

....

....

....

SECOND TRIMESTER

95
DAYS
TO GO

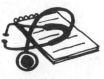

Are you in a group practice and do you
hate one of the doctors? And are you sure
you're going to get him when it's time to deliver?
Short of a scheduled C-section, which is a bit
extreme, it's a lot like Russian roulette.
Look at the bright side. If you hate the doctor,
you'll have very few compunctions about
screaming at him in the delivery room,
when doctors make their guest appearances.
Worry more about the nurses; they'll be with
you every step of the way, and by the end
are often honorary Girlfriends.

N O T E S : ....
....
....
....
....
....

SECOND TRIMESTER

94
DAYS
TO GO

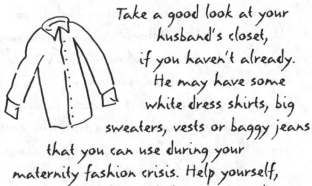

Take a good look at your
husband's closet,
if you haven't already.
He may have some
white dress shirts, big
sweaters, vests or baggy jeans
that you can use during your
maternity fashion crisis. Help yourself,
but don't freak out if they're too tight.

NOTES: ....
....
....
....
....
....

THIRD TRIMESTER

93
DAYS
TO GO

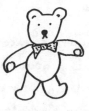

Has it dawned on you yet
that no matter how hard it is
to have this baby inside you,
the job will only get harder
when it comes out?

N O T E S: ....

....

....

....

....

....

THIRD TRIMESTER

Thanks to modern science and age-old
curiosity, there is a good chance that you
already know the gender of your baby.
If it's a boy, your immediate obsession should
now be CIRCUMCISION (or not).
You can't start sharing your concerns
and fears with your husband a minute too soon.
I guarantee, this is one aspect of pregnancy
that is certain to get his attention
and keep it for a nice long time.

N O T E S: ....
....
....
....
....
....

3-19
DATE

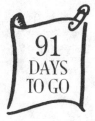

91
DAYS
TO GO

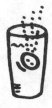

Heartburn does not mean that your baby
will be born with lots of hair.
You can have heartburn so bad that you
spit fire, and your baby can still come out as
bald as Uncle Fester. This condition gets
progressively worse as the baby pushes
open your esophagus. Remember, keep those
antacids handy. They work better than
a fire extinguisher.

NOTES: ....
....
....
....
....
....

THIRD TRIMESTER

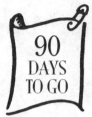

90
DAYS
TO GO

Feeling a little funky? Buy yourself
two or three of those tabloid magazines
and cut out unattractive
photos of pregnant celebrities.
Tape them to your bathroom mirror
for easy reference.

NOTES: ....

....

....

....

....

....

THIRD TRIMESTER

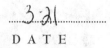

89
DAYS
TO GO

Do you have the sneaking suspicion that you
are getting a crush on your obstetrician? This is
quite common, particularly when your o.b. is a
man. Think about it, he is one of the few people
left on this earth who still seems interested in
how you feel. He is also the only thing that
stands between you and what you secretly believe
is certain death because you know that labor
and delivery survival does not lie in focus
objects, funny breathing or your husband
rolling tennis balls on your lower back.

N O T E S : ....
....
....
....
....
....

THIRD TRIMESTER

88
DAYS
TO GO

........3-22........
D A T E

It may be impossible for you to fully grasp at this
juncture in your life, but right now it is ridiculous
for you to make any informed decisions regarding
vaginal births vs. C-sections, pain medication vs.
relaxation techniques or rooming-in vs. leaving the
baby in the hospital nursery while you sleep. You
haven't a clue yet about how you will feel or what
surprises labor and delivery have in store for you.
Whatever you do, don't expect your experience to be
anything like your prepared childbirth teacher
describes (she doesn't want to alarm you) or
like you've seen on TV, because those shows are
invariably written by childless bachelors.

N O T E S : ....
....
....
....
....

87 DAYS TO GO

You should start thinking now about who you want to go to the hospital with you. Of course, your mate should be at the top of the list, but you might want to invite your mother, sister or Girlfriend. You see, labor often lasts a very long time, and after a few hours husbands tend to annoy their contracting wives.

Almost every woman in deep labor pauses mid-contraction at some point to yell accusingly, "You did this to me!" or "Stop breathing around me; I can't stand the turbulence."

This is a good time for Dad to get a cup of coffee and have the womenfolk step in for a while.

N O T E S: ....
....
....
....
....
....

.......3·24.......
DATE

86
DAYS
TO GO

Boy? girl?

"You're carrying so high, it must be a boy."
"You're positively glowing, it must be a girl."
You may have noticed by now that guessing the
gender of your baby is a favorite hobby for the
public at large. Just wait until someone talks you
into lying on your back while they dangle your
wedding band from a piece of thread over your
belly. If it moves in a clockwise manner, you're
having one sex, and if it moves counterclockwise,
you're having the other. I guess if it moves in a
figure eight, you're having an ice-skater.

NOTES: ....

....

....

....

....

....

THIRD TRIMESTER

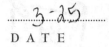

..........**3-25**..........
DATE

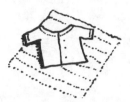

85 DAYS TO GO

Consider registering at a baby store, like brides do at department stores. If someone gives you a baby shower, the guests will appreciate the suggestions and it will help protect you from receiving fifteen darling little cardigan sweaters with matching blankets. After the baby is born, have a few of your close friends spread the word that you're registered, because there is nothing worse than having someone else pick out your diaper bag.

NOTES:..
....
....
....
....
....

THIRD TRIMESTER

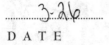

84
DAYS
TO GO

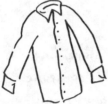

It's time for a detached appraisal of your wardrobe. Those cute little dresses that you have been living in may now be so short in front from your protruding tummy and so long in back from your pregnant swayback that you look like you're tipping over. Same thing applies to tunics, sweaters and T-shirts. Either restrict your wardrobe to long dresses or commit to maternity clothes from here on in. Trust me.

N O T E S: ....

....

....

....

....

....

THIRD TRIMESTER

83
DAYS
TO GO

3-27
D A T E

You have probably received enough unsolicited advice to drive you mad. Don't people understand—pregnancy alone can inspire madness?
Here are a few things to keep in mind:

1. Never believe anything a man tells you (unless he is an obstetrician). He doesn't have a uterus. He has never directly experienced PMS, let alone labor.

2. Keep in mind that most women were high on pain medication when they delivered their babies, so they might not remember the event with great accuracy.

3. Situations that are routine to doctors seem like matters of life and death to first-time parents.

N O T E S : ....
....
....
....
....
....

THIRD TRIMESTER

82
DAYS
TO GO

Let's be grown-ups here for a moment, OK?
Toward the end of your pregnancy, you may learn
that every single thing does not necessarily go
according to the maternity plan you have lovingly
and optimistically concocted. For example, you
might be put on bed rest for a while, or the baby
might be stubbornly staying in the breach position,
or maybe your blood pressure is getting a little
higher than you and your doctor would like.

This is not the time to be a big baby. Just do
what the doctor tells you and stop pouting.
This happens to a lot of us. Remember, you're
still going to end up with a perfect baby.

N O T E S: ....

....

....

....

....

....

THIRD TRIMESTER

Try not to sit in one position too long.
Long car rides, sitting at a desk or parking
yourself in front of a TV can nearly stop the
blood in your legs from circulating back to your
heart if you don't move around every so often.
Imagine holding a bowling ball in your lap for
a couple of hours. Same concept.

Get up and stretch at least once an hour. You
can always use this opportunity to go potty.

N O T E S : ....
....
....
....
....
....

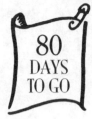

80
DAYS
TO GO

Let's talk about hemorrhoids. These are, for you blessedly uninitiated, little lumps in and around the anus created by blood vessels pooling up and herniating. They are particularly popular among pregnant women and new mommies.

If not for pregnancy, you might have lived your entire life blissfully ignorant of these little grape clusters in your tushie. Between your growing baby cutting off your circulation, not to mention your pushing too hard when constipated, and labor, it's hard to avoid this painful humiliation.

P.S. They go away eventually, only to flare up occasionally or with your next pregnancy.

NOTES: ....

....

....

....

....

....

3.31
DATE

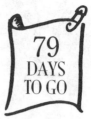

79
DAYS
TO GO

It may be a little over the top to play classical music near your pregnant belly or for your husband to read the classics to it, but babies really do hear you from inside the womb. Just watch after the baby is born; it will quiet to hear Mommy's or Daddy's voice. Of course, it will get to know your voices throughout your entire pregnancy as it eavesdrops on all nearby conversations, whether you are speaking directly to the little sweetie or not. Consider this an inkling of what you have to look forward to as a parent.

NOTES:

THIRD TRIMESTER

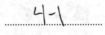
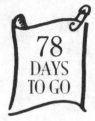

78
DAYS
TO GO

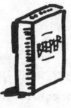

Buy or rent a beeper for your mate. Both of you
will be understandably nervous about labor starting
and your being unable to reach him, especially
in this era of voice mail and other nonhuman
impediments to telephone communication.
Go ahead and test him with a false alarm, but
only ONCE. Sure it will scare the hell out of him,
buy hey, we're all scared, so beep away (ONCE!).

N O T E S : ....
....
....
....
....
....

THIRD TRIMESTER

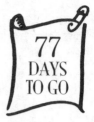

77
DAYS
TO GO

The male population is easily divided into two
camps: those who are aroused by big pregnant
women, and those who are scared to death by
them. You and your partner are probably right now
in the midst of discovering into which category he
falls. Some guys love the luscious ripeness of a
gestating woman, and others find it problematic
having sex with someone who now outweighs
them. Don't worry about it. Either you will become
the sunshine of his life or you and your vibrator
are about to start a meaningful relationship.

N O T E S: ....
....
....
....
....
....

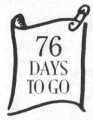

76
DAYS
TO GO

Jade

Try to decide on the baby's name before delivery. Labor is not a good time to make any important decisions. I'll never understand people who say they want to see the baby first; if that was the case, the top names would be E.T. and Kojak.

Jessica

Jeremy

Jamie

NOTES: ....
....
....
....
....
....

4-4

DATE

75
DAYS
TO GO

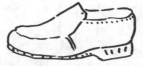

Unless you live in Polynesia, avoid the temptation to wear sandals to relieve the water retention in your sad little feet, especially if it's winter. There must be a loafer or sneaker out there somewhere that you fit into without feeling like one of Cinderella's wicked stepsisters. Fat, swollen feet are rarely attractive and should be hidden at all costs.

NOTES: ....
....
....
....
....
....

THIRD TRIMESTER

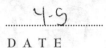
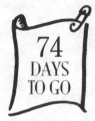

74
DAYS
TO GO

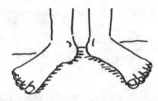

Don't forget to wash your feet and cut
your toenails regularly. Out of sight,
out of mind applies in the personal
hygiene department, and you probably
haven't seen your feet in weeks.

N O T E S : ....

....

....

....

....

....

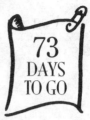

73 DAYS TO GO

Does it come as any surprise that, like several of your other organs, your bowels have turned against you in your time of need? Yes, we're talking about constipation. The first step toward a cure is to up your water and fiber intake. Then check with your doctor to ask whether an iron supplement in your prenatal vitamins could be contributing to the logjam. While you have him or her on the line, you might also ask request a suggestion for a stool softener. In the meantime, pay attention to the muscles you use to have a "movement" because they are the same ones you'll use to deliver the baby. Bet nobody ever told you that before!

N O T E S: ....
....
....
....
....
....

THIRD TRIMESTER

......4-7......
DATE

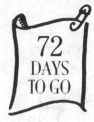

72
DAYS
TO GO

There is really no use making up dream
labor scenarios, whether they include flawless
Lamaze breathing or drugs on demand,
because this experience is nothing if not surprising.
If you get too hooked on a preconceived
(no pun intended) notion of a "perfect" way
for your child to enter this world, you're setting
a standard that is rigid, judgmental and
uninformed. Remember, no matter whether you
deliver your child alone in a rice paddy or receive
it via Federal Express, it is a "perfect" delivery.

N O T E S : ....
....
....
....
....
....

THIRD TRIMESTER

<u>4 - 8</u>

DATE

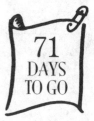

71
DAYS
TO GO

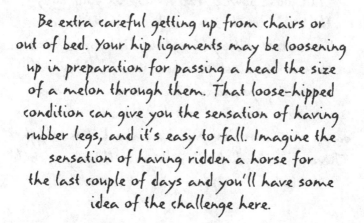

Be extra careful getting up from chairs or
out of bed. Your hip ligaments may be loosening
up in preparation for passing a head the size
of a melon through them. That loose-hipped
condition can give you the sensation of having
rubber legs, and it's easy to fall. Imagine the
sensation of having ridden a horse for
the last couple of days and you'll have some
idea of the challenge here.

NOTES:...
....
....
....
....
....

THIRD TRIMESTER

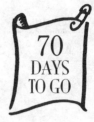

70
DAYS
TO GO

Put loose powder everywhere on your body
that skin touches skin. This could take some
time. Start with your substantial upper arms;
they rub against your breasts and sides with
every step you take. Then move on to where
your breasts rest on your belly; that's usually as
damp as the tropics. And how about those thighs?
There is so much friction between them you could
light a campfire without a match.

N O T E S : ....
....
....
....
....
....

THIRD TRIMESTER

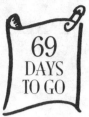

69
DAYS
TO GO

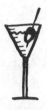

Aren't parties a bore now? No sexy
little black dresses, no wine or salty margaritas.
Even the hors d'oeuvres give you heartburn.
You will now learn something that every
practicing member of a twelve-step program
already knows: Drunk people are incredibly
tiresome if you're not one of them.

The Girlfriends' suggestion? Stay home and
catch up on some sleep.

NOTES:..
....
....
....
....
....

THIRD TRIMESTER

68 DAYS TO GO

Somewhere between 15 and 30 percent of all American deliveries are by cesarean section, depending on your doctor and the hospital in which you deliver. This is a fact, not a judgment, since I think any relatively painless method of giving birth is just swell, but it is an indication that you should be flexible in your expectations about what lies ahead of you. There is a fairly good chance that your baby will not emerge after one hour of hee-hee breathing and a couple of good pushes. You will be the hero no matter what happens and your baby will be spectacular and, really, isn't that all that matters?

NOTES: ....
....
....
....
....
....

THIRD TRIMESTER

67
DAYS
TO GO

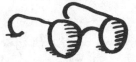

If you wear contact lenses, you may find that the
prescription seems off. There is so much water
being retained in your body and your blood vessels
are so dilated that your eyeballs can actually
change shape enough to fuzz up your vision.
Don't throw your contacts away, however, because
they will fit again after the baby is born.
Unlike your feet and other unmentionable body
parts, your eyes will go back to normal.

N O T E S:...

....

....

....

....

....

THIRD TRIMESTER

66
DAYS
TO GO

Beware of the Pregnancy Police, Girlfriend. These are the folks who feel obligated to look into your grocery cart and comment if you have diet soda or something with preservatives in it. They also park themselves in airports near the security checks to make sure you don't walk through the metal detectors. Their favorite haunts, however, are restaurants where they lie in wait for a pregnant woman to sip some wine. Then they pounce on her, spewing factoids about fetal alcohol syndrome. These people are not well-intentioned, they are just busybodies and deserve to be ignored.

NOTES: ....
....
....
....
....
....

THIRD TRIMESTER

65
DAYS
TO GO

Some of you already know by this time that you are going to have a C-section. Perhaps the baby is really big, or you have a little herpes outbreak or some other reason why a vaginal birth isn't going to work out.

C-sections, particularly those that are scheduled, can be at least as rewarding and thrilling as vaginal births. There is something wonderful about knowing when your baby is coming. You can drive relatively calmly to the hospital, you will be perfectly groomed <u>and</u> you get to keep the vagina of a teenager.

NOTES:..
....
....
....
....
....

THIRD TRIMESTER

64
DAYS
TO GO

Prepare a list of names and phone numbers of the people you want your husband to call after the baby is born, and pack it in your suitcase. He will be delirious and certainly won't have a phone book, and you will probably be eating or sleeping by this time.

The rule of thumb regarding phone calls is this: Call all immediate relatives and close friends who've had kids as soon as possible, day or night. Call all childless friends before 10 p.m. or after 9 a.m.; they may not be able to comprehend the sheer miraculousness of the event if they are awakened from a deep sleep.

N O T E S : ....
....
....
....
....
....

63
DAYS
TO GO

Beg a mommy Girlfriend to accompany you
and your husband to a baby store when
you're ready to buy furniture and other equally
mystifying infant necessities.
YOU DON'T NEED EVERYTHING ON THE
SHOWROOM FLOOR,
and you'll want a more disinterested party
than the salesperson to guide you. Short of
delivery itself, this can be one of the
scariest aspects of pregnancy
(and that's <u>before</u> you get the bill!).

NOTES: ....
....
....
....
....
....

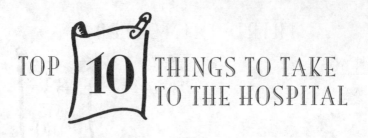

TOP **10** THINGS TO TAKE TO THE HOSPITAL

10. YOUR HUSBAND. HE'S NOT ESSENTIAL, BUT IT'S NICE TO HAVE SOMEONE TO BLAME FOR YOUR MISERY. A GIRLFRIEND MIGHT BE FUN TO GIVE YOUR HUSBAND A CAFETERIA BREAK EVERY NOW AND THEN.

9. LIP BALM. EVEN THOUGH IT'S YOUR OTHER LIPS THAT ARE SEEING ALL THE ACTION DURING DELIVERY, THE LIPS ON YOUR MOUTH TEND TO GET VERY DRY, ESPECIALLY IF YOU TRY ANY EXOTIC BREATHING TECHNIQUES.

8. YOUR OWN BED PILLOWS IN OLD PILLOWCASES. NOT ONLY ARE THEY INFINITELY MORE COMFORTABLE THAN HOSPITAL-ISSUE, THEY SMELL LIKE HOME AND THAT CAN BE A COMFORT AMIDST ALL THE BETADINE AROMAS IN A LABOR AND DELIVERY ROOM.

7. CAMERAS, BOTH VIDEO AND STILL, WITH EXTRA FILM FOR BOTH. MAKE SURE THAT YOU HAVE CHARGED THE VIDEO CAM'S BATTERIES AND HAVE BROUGHT AN EXTRA BECAUSE YOU MAY USE UP ALL YOUR POWER BEFORE THE GUEST OF HONOR ARRIVES.

6. EXTRA SOCKS. FOOTSIES GET COLD DURING LABOR. THE DOCTOR WILL LET YOU KEEP THEM ON THROUGH DELIVERY, TOO, BUT THEY MAY GET A LITTLE BLOODY AT THAT POINT, SO HAVE SEVERAL PAIRS TO REPLACE THEM AS NEEDED.

5. FOOD AND WATER. SOME GRANOLA BARS OR TRAIL MIX, MAYBE SOME POPCORN, CAN COME IN VERY HANDY AFTER DELIVERY WHEN YOU'RE STARVING, BUT THE HOSPITAL'S NOT SERVING. BOTTLED WATER IS ALWAYS TASTIER THAN THE STUFF THEY PUT IN THE LITTLE PLASTIC PITCHER ON YOUR BEDSIDE TABLE.

4. YOUR GLASSES, IF YOU USUALLY WEAR CONTACTS. A COUPLE GOOD PUSHES CAN SEND CONTACTS FLYING ACROSS THE ROOM, BUT YOU MAY WANT TO GET A GOOD LOOK AT THE BABY WHEN IT COMES.

3. MATERNITY CLOTHES TO WEAR HOME FROM THE HOSPITAL. SORRY, BUT YOU WILL STILL BE FAT. BESIDES, YOU WILL NEED THE GIGANTIC PANTIES TO HOLD THE MANY SANITARY PADS YOU WILL BE WEARING FOR THE NEXT FEW DAYS. THIS INCLUDES A NURSING BRA IF YOU INTEND TO GIVE THAT A TRY.

2. YOUR OWN TOILETRIES, INCLUDING SHAMPOO, SOAP, LOTION AND TOOTHPASTE. OF CRITICAL IMPORTANCE ARE MAKEUP AND YOUR OWN BLOW-DRYER; REMEMBER, IT'S A PHOTO FREE-FOR-ALL ONCE THE BABY ARRIVES.

1. A LIST OF NAMES AND PHONE NUMBERS IN ORDER OF IMPORTANCE AND A TELEPHONE CALLING CARD SO YOUR HUSBAND CAN USE THE PAY PHONES WITHOUT CARRYING MORE CHANGE THAN A SLOT MACHINE ATTENDANT.

THIRD TRIMESTER

62 DAYS TO GO

You may have noticed a yellowish liquid
leaking from your breasts when you squeeze them
(don't we all spend our free time squeezing
our own breasts?). If you have, congratulations,
you are making colostrum, the premilk food
nursed babies eat for the first couple of days
of life. If your squeezing isn't yielding anything,
or if you just prefer not to squeeze, don't fret;
the colostrum is in there anyway.

NOTES: ....

....

....

....

....

....

4-18
_____

DATE

61
DAYS
TO GO

Should you nurse? Our best answer is this: Don't do it unless you really want to. This is not something you must try just because your Lamaze teacher told you to. Here is another area in which you have the Girlfriends' full understanding and support if you ignore all societal pressure and do what is specifically right for you and your unique circumstances. Nursing is great. For some people, it is better than orgasm and lasts longer. But you can live a full and wonderful life never having hung one single human from your breasts. If you don't believe me, just ask your mother.

NOTES:..
....
....
....
....
....

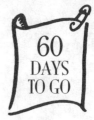

60
DAYS
TO GO

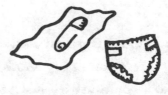

The diaper debate rages on: cloth or disposable?
Your choice here will not affect your
overall grade in Motherhood 101, so relax.
Here's our general guideline: If you live in
an arid area that is prone to droughts,
use disposables because you won't waste water
washing them. If you live near Niagara Falls
or in a rain forest, use cloth and
keep the landfill dumping to a minimum.
There, wasn't that easy?

N O T E S: ....
....
....
....
....
....

THIRD TRIMESTER

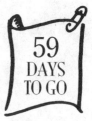

59
DAYS
TO GO

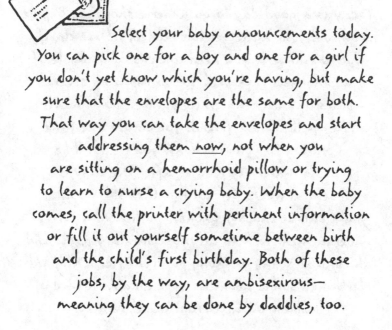

        Select your baby announcements today.
You can pick one for a boy and one for a girl if
you don't yet know which you're having, but make
sure that the envelopes are the same for both.
That way you can take the envelopes and start
        addressing them _now_, not when you
    are sitting on a hemorrhoid pillow or trying
to learn to nurse a crying baby. When the baby
comes, call the printer with pertinent information
or fill it out yourself sometime between birth
and the child's first birthday. Both of these
        jobs, by the way, are ambisexirous—
    meaning they can be done by daddies, too.

N O T E S: ....
....
....
....
....
....

THIRD TRIMESTER

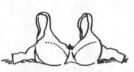

Today is a good day to go lingerie shopping. Before you and your mate get too excited, let me clarify that the lingerie you need consists of a couple of nursing bras with peek-a-boo cups and several pairs of cheap maternity panties. Don't howl! They will be your friends for quite some time. Contrary to your illusions, you will still be using maternity panties after the baby is several weeks (if not months) old. First, you'll still be chubby; second, you'll need a serious undergarment to hold all those sanitary pads; and third, a G-string or thong panties after a vaginal birth will sound about as appealing as a wad of bubble gum after root canal surgery.

NOTES:...
....
....
....
....
....

4-22
<u>...............................</u>

D A T E

57
DAYS
TO GO

Do not insist that your mate cut the
umbilical cord or take a long and loving
look at the placenta, even though your doctor
will probably offer both opportunities.
If he wants to, fine. If his upper lip gets sweaty
at the suggestion, allow him to decline.
This is no time to ruin the moment with
arguments and disappointments. Save them
for the first day home from the hospital.

N O T E S: ....
....
....
....
....
....

4-23
....

D A T E

56
DAYS
TO GO

Upsetting stories abound about laboring women being given enemas before delivery. I would rather carry that baby in utero for the rest of my life than have an enema.

The great news is this is one indignity you don't have to endure. In fact, several of my Girlfriends were never even offered the chance to decline; nobody suggested it to them. I think there used to be a worry that if you pushed hard to get the baby out, some poopoo would come out, too. Well, that does indeed happen, but since they don't come out of the same opening, nobody really cares. And neither should you.

N O T E S:...
....
....
....
....
....

THIRD TRIMESTER

55
DAYS
TO GO

All seriously pregnant women
get the desperate urge to pee and
frantically run to the bathroom, only
to find that a tiny trickle comes out
when they sit down. If you think that you have
had pregnancy up to here, just pause to think
how your little pancake of a bladder must
be feeling about now.

NOTES: ....
....
....
....
....
....

4-25

D A T E

54
DAYS
TO GO

You should be looking into available
"prepared childbirth" classes right about now.
You will get a big kick out of them at first,
then learn to feel trapped and pressured by
them. Your husband will dislike them at
the beginning and be openly hostile by the end...
but they're as much a part of
pregnancy as stretch marks.

N O T E S: ....

....

....

....

....

....

53
DAYS
TO GO

Don't let the Girlfriends' affection for epidurals make you think that we don't believe in prepared childbirth classes.

First of all, pain avoidance through controlled breathing is a wonderful skill to have, especially for bikini waxes or any dental procedure where the dentist says, "This will only sting for a minute." Second, it can be fun to get in a room full of other butterballs...and third, classes can be fulfilling for those people who just can't see enough grainy movies of complete strangers giving birth.

NOTES:..
....
....
....
....
....

THIRD TRIMESTER

52
DAYS
TO GO

Many of us Girlfriends suffered the ultimate
indignity of having our belly buttons pop out during
our last few weeks of pregnancy. It can make a
very noticeable bump, even through a blouse or
dress, and you will panic if someone comes toward
you with an outstretched hand ready to pat your
belly. Girlfriends' tip: Put a thick Band-Aid over
your belly button and then wear maternity panty
hose whenever you leave your house. That ought
to flatten things out sufficiently.

N O T E S: ....
....
....
....
....
....

THIRD TRIMESTER

51
DAYS
TO GO

You may feel jumpy now that labor
and delivery are within spitting distance.
Take a deep breath and try to relax.
Oh, we forgot, you can't take deep breaths
anymore. In fact, you're so full of baby
that you are claustrophobic.
We promise you will get immediate
relief the instant the baby appears.

NOTES:

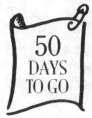

50
DAYS
TO GO

Here is another phrase for your
pregnancy vocabulary: "vagina farts."
These little emissions occur when the baby is
large, head down, and pressing against your
cervix so hard that it feels like your
labia are down around your knees.

Walking, bending over, lifting—whatever—work
like a bellows, sucking in and puffing out little
bubbles of air, unfortunately accompanied by
raspberry sounds. Just act shocked and look
around as if wondering what boor had
the gall to make such a noise.

N O T E S: ....
....
....
....
....
....

THIRD TRIMESTER

49 DAYS TO GO

It's getting harder and harder to eat now. Your stomach is smashed up flat as a pancake under your rib cage, and even though you are constantly hungry, you are full after two bites.

Think of yourself as a hummingbird (don't laugh, I could have said cow), and just take sips (or graze) throughout the entire day. You may even lose a pound or two right before delivery as your appetite continues to shrink. Don't worry, you'll eat like a lumberjack as soon as your baby has been taken to the hospital nursery and you have flagged down a nurse (or maybe your husband!) to bring you some food.

N O T E S : ....

....

....

....

....

....

48
DAYS
TO GO

Sleeping is getting harder and harder
with every week, right? Some hopeless
optimists (usually childless) will tell you
that this is nature's way of getting you
used to the scarcity of sleep you will
experience as a new mother. What a crock!
That's like saying dieting prepares
you for starvation.

You aren't sleeping because there is only room
for one of you in this body, pardner.

N O T E S: ....
....
....
....
....
....

THIRD TRIMESTER

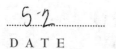

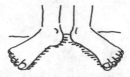

Pedicures should be particularly important to you now. Think about it...what part of your body will be closest to your obstetrician's face during check-ups and delivery? WRONG!!! I'm talking about your feet. You may not notice them yourself at this point, hidden as they are by your belly, but don't get negligent about this critical area of grooming.

If you have the extra time and money, indulge in a professional pedicure. First of all, you probably can't reach your toes yourself; and, second, your bloated feet could use a massage.

N O T E S : ....

....

....

....

....

....

TOP 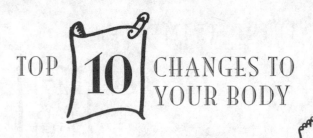 10 CHANGES TO YOUR BODY

10. YOUR FEET ARE SWOLLEN AND LARGER, AND THE BAD NEWS IS THAT THEY MAY PERMANENTLY GROW AN EXTRA SHOE SIZE. THE GOOD NEWS IS THAT IT DOESN'T HAPPEN WITH EACH SUBSEQUENT BIRTH.

9. YOUR DIGESTIVE SYSTEM IS SLIGHTLY DYSFUNCTIONAL. BETWEEN GAS AND HEARTBURN, YOU CAN HARDLY STAND TO BE AROUND YOURSELF.

8. YOU WILL BE CHANGING COLORS IN ALL SORTS OF PLACES, NOT JUST TURNING GREEN. FROM YOUR NIPPLES TO YOUR LABIA, THERE'S NO TELLING WHERE THIS WILL TURN UP.

7. FLASHING BACK TO PUBERTY? IT'S JUST PREGNANCY PIMPLES. YOUR COMPLEXION, LIKE THE REST OF YOUR BODY, MAY CHANGE COLOR AND BECOME BLOTCHY TO BOOT. IF YOU'RE ONE OF THE "LUCKY" ONES,

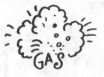
GAS

YOU MAY GET TINY FLAPS OF EXTRA SKIN, USUALLY UNDER YOUR ARM OR ON THE EYELID.

6. TWO WORDS: STRETCH MARKS. WE HAVE NO WORDS OF WISDOM, JUST ANOTHER THING TO BLAME YOUR MOTHER FOR— THEY'RE HEREDITARY.

5. LUXURIOUS HAIR AND NAILS—PLAY THEM UP, THEY CAN HIDE A MULTITUDE OF SINS.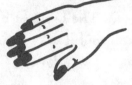

4. YOUR BUTT IS GETTING LARGER. DON'T WORRY, THE BABY'S NOT GROWING THE WRONG WAY, THOUGH IT MAY FEEL LIKE THAT.

3. WATER RETENTION WITH NOWHERE TO DRAIN (IT ALMOST MAKES YOU LONG FOR YOUR PERIOD). YOUR ENTIRE BODY IS PUFFIER, FROM YOUR NOSE TO TOES.

2. BIG BOUNCING BREASTS THAT WILL CONTINUE TO BLOOM ALL NINE (TEN) MONTHS.

1. OVERWHELMING BODILY FUNCTIONS, WITH THE WINNER BEING PEEING. A CLOSE RUNNER-UP IS CONSTIPATION.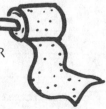

THIRD TRIMESTER

46
DAYS
TO GO

Women approaching their due date are worried sick that they will go into labor and not recognize it. The thought of going to the hospital and being told it was a false alarm becomes the highest form of humiliation imaginable.

Let the Girlfriends reassure you right away that far more humiliating things are in store for you. Even more to the point, consider all trips to the hospital that don't result in the birth of a baby very valuable dress rehearsals for the real opening night (pun intended).

N O T E S : ....
....
....
....
....
....

THIRD TRIMESTER

DATE

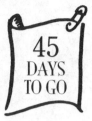

45
DAYS
TO GO

This is just another reminder to keep up with
your Kegels. You may think we are making a
big deal out of something that could turn out
to be a great spoof like being invited to watch
the submarine races or waiting for the salmon
to spawn, but this is real, we promise.
I don't care what you hear to the contrary,
if you don't keep toned in there, your career
as a trampoline artist is history because your
bladder will fail at every bounce.

NOTES: ....
....
....
....
....
....

THIRD TRIMESTER

44
DAYS
TO GO

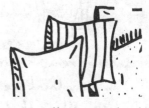

Bring your own pillows to the hospital.
Since it is still traditional for women to spend
a lot of labor in bed, you will definitely prefer
your own fluffy friends to the cardboard
institutional pillows you will be issued.
A less obvious but very important quality your
pillows have is that they smell like home. That
familiar scent and feeling can be immeasurably
reassuring at a time like this.

N O T E S : ....
....
....
....
....
....

THIRD TRIMESTER

43 DAYS TO GO

The arrival of a new baby is the greatest photo opportunity on the planet. You will probably want to record this event both on still film and on video. Guess what? You will be in almost every picture!

If you want to look at these pictures in years to come without humiliation, consider applying light, waterproof makeup and washing and styling your hair before checking into the hospital. Trust me, as superficial as this advice may sound today, you will thank me with flowers and gifts when your pictures come back from the developers. If your makeup has run and smeared, my number is unlisted.

N O T E S: ....
....
....
....
....
....

THIRD TRIMESTER

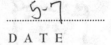

42
DAYS
TO GO

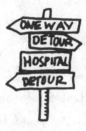

You and your mate should take a practice run
to the hospital sometime soon. Pick your route
and stick to it. One major cause of delivery
panic is when there are too many options and
a rational decision must be made. It is wise to
eliminate all multiple-choice questions in areas
related to this baby as soon as possible.

N O T E S: ....

....

....

....

....

....

41
DAYS
TO GO

You must have a good car seat.
It is against the law in most states for
a hospital to release a baby until you have shown
them that you have a car seat ready for it. This is
a good rule, not only because it keeps the baby safe
for the ride home, but it's a good way of identify-
ing nincompoop parents who haven't fully adjusted
to their new responsibilities. Since you will probably
need two sizes of car seats during the next four
years of your baby's life, make sure one is the
infant model that snaps into a frame in the
car and snaps out to become a baby carrier.
That way you don't wake the baby moving it from
the car to the house—a crucial feature.

N O T E S : ....
....
....
....
....
....

THIRD TRIMESTER

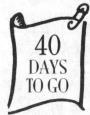

40 DAYS TO GO

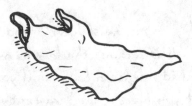

Do not go shopping for a beautiful nightgown
and robe to wear in the hospital after the
baby is born. You will only be in the hospital
for what will seem like minutes, and you will
still be leaking all sorts of yucky stuff that stains.
Save your nightie for your own home, and
bleed all over the hospital's gowns and sheets.
That's what they're charging you for.

NOTES: ....

....

....

....

....

....

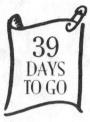

39
DAYS
TO GO

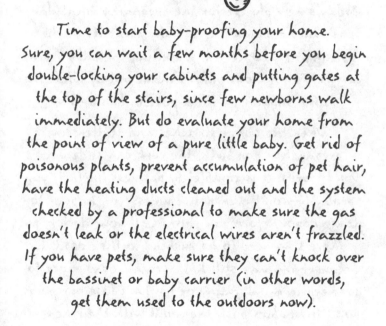

Time to start baby-proofing your home.
Sure, you can wait a few months before you begin
double-locking your cabinets and putting gates at
the top of the stairs, since few newborns walk
immediately. But do evaluate your home from
the point of view of a pure little baby. Get rid of
poisonous plants, prevent accumulation of pet hair,
have the heating ducts cleaned out and the system
checked by a professional to make sure the gas
doesn't leak or the electrical wires aren't frazzled.
If you have pets, make sure they can't knock over
the bassinet or baby carrier (in other words,
get them used to the outdoors now).

N O T E S: ....
....
....
....
....
....

5-11

D A T E

38
DAYS
TO GO

Today's new phrase for the pregnancy vocabulary is <u>mucous plug</u>. This squishy cork sits in the opening of your cervix, protecting the baby from germs. The mucous plug is made out of what the name suggests, with a pinkish blood color.

When the cervix stretches and flattens in preparation for birth, the cork can slide out. Don't worry, it is completely painless. In fact, you probably won't even notice unless you happen to glance down before you flush. Call your doctor, but there's no need to go rushing to the hospital because you may still have several days more to go. Keep in mind, many of us don't lose our plugs until the babies push them out with their heads.

N O T E S: ....
....
....
....
....
....

THIRD TRIMESTER

37
DAYS
TO GO

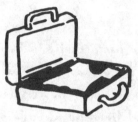

It's time to pack your bag now, even if you swear it's too soon. Remember, if you go into labor before you've packed, your husband will be left with that job. Can't you just see him walking into the hospital with a shopping bag under his arm filled with something sleeveless, too-tight jeans, and no underwear or deodorant?

NOTES: ....
....
....
....
....
....

THIRD TRIMESTER

36
DAYS
TO GO

It is easier for a turtle to turn from its back to its belly than for a very pregnant woman to roll over in her sleep. Buy or borrow one of those total body pillows to use until D day. Hold on to it like it's a crocodile and you're Paul Hogan. Give a big rock-and-roll motion to get the momentum necessary to turn the two of you over. Your husband may feel a little alienated. Then again, he may be relieved that your needs are being met by something other than him.

N O T E S: ....
....
....
....
....

THIRD TRIMESTER

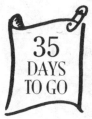

35
DAYS
TO GO

We know you know this, but it bears
repeating right about now. Your due date is
nothing more than an estimation. Very few
butterballs actually pop on that very date, and
you probably won't either. Try not to drive
yourself crazy expecting that day to bring relief
from this never-ending condition of pregnancy,
because odds are that you will be early and caught
off-guard, or late and pissed off.

NOTES:..
....
....
....
....
....

5-15
....

D A T E

34
DAYS
TO GO

If you intend to nurse your baby, it's about time for you to look into renting an electric breast pump. All nursing mothers with lives know that a stock of pumped milk in the freezer is better than money in the bank. It gives them freedom to take a nap or go to the grocery store without fearing that their little darling will starve or be forced to move on to formula.

Look in the yellow pages or ask your doctor for a number.

N O T E S:...
....
....
....
....
....

THIRD TRIMESTER

33
DAYS
TO GO

This is a very stressful time for most husbands. They have watched enough old movies to know that babies arrive with great unpredictability, with the men invariably panicking and speeding off into the night, leaving the laboring mother standing in the driveway beside her little suitcase.

He's like a child who knows that something is hiding somewhere in the house and he has no idea what closet it will pop out of. Help the poor guy out and remind him that babies, especially first babies, usually give plenty of warning before exploding into our world.

N O T E S: ....
....
....
....
....
....

THIRD TRIMESTER

DATE

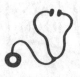

32 DAYS TO GO

Uh-oh! The baby doesn't seem to be moving as often or as vigorously. You imagine the very worst, but your fear has you too paralyzed to even call the doctor.

The baby is fine! As it gets bigger, there is less room for it to get a good kick in, and as it settles head-down in preparation for birth, it really feels jammed.

Do us all a favor and call your doctor immediately—not because something is wrong, but because they will have you come in and check you out. It will be a tremendous relief for everyone, particularly those who live with you.

NOTES:..
....
....
....
....
....

THIRD TRIMESTER

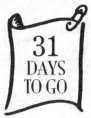

✓ CheckUp

Sometime near your due date, your doctor
may give you something called a "non-stress test."
This refers to the baby's not being stressed—
<u>you</u> are stressed by nearly everything
these days. This test consists of your lying
down with a fetal monitor around your belly.
This will record your baby's heart rate
when it moves and show whether it is strong
and ready to blast into this world.

NOTES:...
....
....
....
....
....

THIRD TRIMESTER

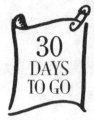

30
DAYS
TO GO

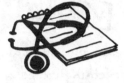

About now, the internal exams begin again.
The doctor will be looking inside you for
signs of dilation and effacement. You will
be looking for the doctor, who will doubtless
be carrying on a conversation with you,
and you won't be able to see him
or her because your belly completely
blocks your line of vision.

N O T E S: ....

....

....

....

....

....

THIRD TRIMESTER

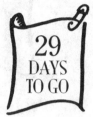

29 DAYS TO GO

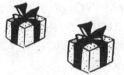

Now is a good time for a baby shower
if you intend to have one. You have time to kill,
you deserve a major distraction and you can
spend the next few days and weeks washing
the clothes in Dreft or decorating the nursery
with the adorable stuff you have received.

N O T E S: ....
....
....
....
....
....

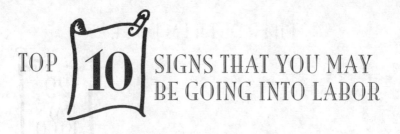

TOP **10** SIGNS THAT YOU MAY BE GOING INTO LABOR

10. DIARRHEA OR OTHER FLU-LIKE SYMPTOMS. YOUR BODY MAY DO SOME SERIOUS SPRING CLEANING OF ITS OWN IN ANTICIPATION OF THE BABY'S ARRIVAL.

9. FRENZIED, OBSESSIVE CLEANING AND ORGANIZING. IF YOU GET UP AT 2 A.M. WITH AN IRRESISTIBLE NEED TO SEW NAME LABELS IN THE BABY'S UNDER-SHIRTS, YOU MAY BE ABOUT TO POP.

8. YOU'VE STOPPED EATING. FEW THINGS LOOK APPETIZING, AND NOTHING IS REALLY DIGESTING AT THIS POINT. ICE CUBES HAVE BECOME YOUR MEAL OF CHOICE.

7. YOU JUST FOUND A SLIMY, BLOODY HUNK OF MUCOUS IN YOUR PANTIES OR IN THE TOILET. (YOUR MUCOUS PLUG CAN COME OUT WHEN YOU START DILATING AND EFFACING.)

6. YOU ARE WETTING YOUR PANTS, AND YOU CAN'T STOP (A SIGN THAT THE SAC OF AMNIOTIC FLUID HAS BURST, OR YOUR "WATER HAS BROKEN").

5. YOUR HAIR IS DIRTY, YOU HAVEN'T DONE LAUNDRY IN TEN DAYS AND THE CAR NEEDS GAS. GUARANTEED TO GO INTO LABOR TONIGHT.

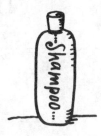

4. YOUR LOWER BACK HURTS SO MUCH YOU WOULD SWEAR YOU'VE BEEN LIFTING APPLIANCES IN YOUR SLEEP.

3. YOU JUST GOT AN INTERNAL EXAM, AND THE DOCTOR TOLD YOU WHAT COLOR THE BABY'S

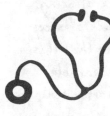

HAIR IS. (JUST KIDDING THERE, GIRLFRIEND, BUT HE OR SHE MIGHT HAVE TOLD YOU THAT YOU ARE TWO OR THREE CENTIMETERS DILATED AND COMPLETELY EFFACED.)

2. YOU ARE EXPERIENCING MENSTRUAL-LIKE CRAMPS SO COMPELLING THAT YOU NOT ONLY CAN'T TALK DURING ONE, BUT YOU CAN'T LISTEN EITHER AND YOU THREATEN TO KILL ANYONE WHO CHATTERS TO YOU WHILE YOU QUAKE.

1. YOU ARE IN A HOSPITAL BED WATCHING WHEEL OF FORTUNE WITH AN INTRAVENOUS DRIP OF LABOR-INDUCING PITOCIN FLOWING THROUGH YOUR VEINS AND AN EPIDURAL COMFORTABLY NUMBING YOU FROM THE WAIST DOWN.

THIRD TRIMESTER

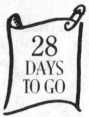

28 DAYS TO GO

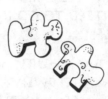

Welcome to Maternity Limbo!
From this time on, you are living in suspended
animation. You're probably sick of being
pregnant and exhausted from lack of sleep
and surplus weight. We all agree that this
"holding pattern" is nearly unbearable.
Don't be shocked if you feel even shorter-tempered
than usual or cry several times a day.
You will make it, Girlfriend, we promise.
Try a thousand-piece jigsaw puzzle or put loose
photos in your albums to distract yourself.

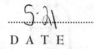

N O T E S: ....
....
....
....
....
....

27
DAYS
TO GO

If your car is equipped with airbags,
always put the baby's car seat
(and the baby, too, when it comes)
in the backseat. It doesn't take too
great an impact to activate the bags,
and the explosion upon opening can
seriously hurt a tiny person.

NOTES:..
....
....
....
....
....

THIRD TRIMESTER

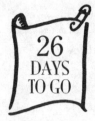

26
DAYS
TO GO

Just when you thought you couldn't
possibly look more pregnant,
you grew some more. At this point,
your belly is no longer a smooth,
rounded protrusion, but something
that seems to have points and corners
where the elbows, feet and knees stick out.
When a pregnant belly looks low and
"squared," you are approaching liftoff.

NOTES:...

....

....

....

....

....

THIRD TRIMESTER

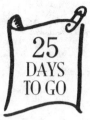

25 DAYS TO GO

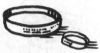

Which mementos of your baby's birth should you save for posterity? Certainly, you must keep the hospital bracelets that the two of you wore, and the pink or blue name cards from the hospital bassinet. Lots of us save the baby blanket with the name of the industrial laundry company on it, and a really big favorite is the knit cap they put on the baby's head as soon as he gets his first shampoo.

More controversial is the belly button stump. We suggest that for preserved body parts, you draw the line at locks of hair and baby teeth.

N O T E S : ....

....

....

....

....

....

THIRD TRIMESTER

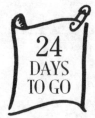

24
DAYS
TO GO

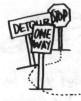

No matter how desperate you may be
for distraction at this point, don't plan any
weekend getaways. Even though you swear
this baby is never coming, it is, and it wants to
come to a hospital that it knows and trusts...
not to the first-aid center in Caesar's Palace.
Stay within a forty-mile radius of the
hospital that has preadmitted you.

N O T E S : ....

....

....

....

....

....

......5-26.........
D A T E

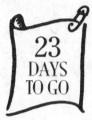

23 DAYS TO GO

Beg, bribe or call your congressman to make sure that you will be able to stay in the hospital for at least 48 hours after delivery. Sure, the food stinks and the pillows are made out of packing materials, but it's filled with doctors and nurses and other people who are sure to know much more about new babies than you do. One of this Girlfriend's most treasured memories was in the middle of the night in the hospital, watching old movies with her brand-new baby. Sheer bliss, especially if someone happens to send you a congratulatory muffin or cookie basket.

N O T E S :...
....
....
....
....
....

THIRD TRIMESTER

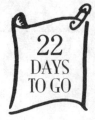

22
DAYS
TO GO

When you feel like your spine just can't
take this pregnancy one more minute,
get down on your hands and knees—
not to pray, although it couldn't hurt—
but to do what are called "cat stretches."
First, slowly curve your back up like a scared cat,
then gently release it into a swayback.
Do this five or ten times to get a little blood
circulating. Then, feel free to lie down
on the floor and take a nap.

N O T E S: ....
....
....
....
....
....

5-28

D A T E

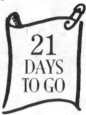

21
DAYS
TO GO

To snip or not to snip. If you have a boy, you will
be asked, before your baby is 24 hours old,
whether you intend to circumcise him. A practice
that has been routine in this country for years
is now being reexamined. Most mothers are
tempted to take the route of the least amount of
discomfort, but most fathers assume that their
son's peepee must look exactly like their peepee.

We suggest you let your husband make this
call since penis care is not within our immediate
area of expertise, and, if you are Jewish, there
really is no use in questioning the divine wisdom
of God and men. Women used to get burned
at the stake for far less.

N O T E S : ....

....

....

....

....

....

<u>5.29</u>

DATE

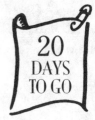

20
DAYS
TO GO

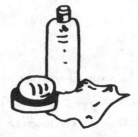

At this point, it must seem to you that you
visit the o.b. every other day. They really
start paying attention when you're this pregnant.
Try to be bathed and groomed for every one
of these visits because if you can't pull it together
for your doctor, you have really lost your grip.
Besides, the other people in the office are looking
to you for inspiration, not to be terrified by
impending motherhood.

NOTES:...
....
....
....
....
....

THIRD TRIMESTER

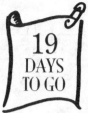

19
DAYS
TO GO

If you have already received baby shower gifts,
write your thank-you notes TODAY. You will
receive more gifts after the baby is born, and if
you get behind now, you will never catch up.
Remember, it will seem like only moments before
you're writing thank-yous for the
holidays, and before you know it,
first birthdays are here
with more gifts
to be acknowledged.

N O T E S: ....
....
....
....
....
....

THIRD TRIMESTER

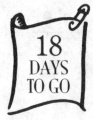

18
DAYS
TO GO

You will be overwhelmed by many, many things in the weeks to come, and one of the important lessons for you to start teaching your husband is that he will be responsible for various things in the near future that normally he would expect you to handle. But you'll have your hands full, literally and figuratively.

P.S. Among the new daddy jobs will be helping you with thank-yous for gifts and flowers and manning the phones. (He does handle a full-time job; he should be able to swing this.)

NOTES:...
....
....
....
....
....

THIRD TRIMESTER

6-1

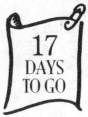

17
DAYS
TO GO

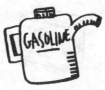

Is there gas in the car?
Never let the tank get below half-empty
from now until your children are married
and gone. Trust us, you will not want to
stop for a fill-up when you're in labor,
nor will you in the future when you
are driving a vomiting six-year-old
to the pediatrician.

N O T E S: ....
....
....
....
....
....

THIRD TRIMESTER

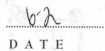
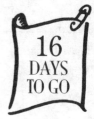

16
DAYS
TO GO

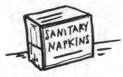

You will have a bloody discharge for weeks
after delivery, whether it was a vaginal or
cesarean birth. I considered investing in a sanitary
pad company (remember, you won't be using
tampons yet) because, in the beginning, I was using
two or three at a time. The flow will change color,
from reddish to brownish to yellowish to gone.
If you notice blood that looks like what comes out
of a cut, rather than menstrual-looking blood,
call the doctor; you might be hemorrhaging.

N O T E S : ....
....
....
....
....
....

THIRD TRIMESTER

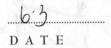
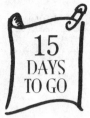

15
DAYS
TO GO

It's never too early to obsess ahead; you will be completely within your rights to demand that all visitors, even your mate should you deem it necessary, wash with antibacterial soap before entering your baby's universe. Some mommies feel that even this is not enough protection (you can't help yourself), and they require guests to wear surgical gowns or drape themselves in a large baby blanket. You are the boss here. You have the right to dip them in hydrogen peroxide as far as we are concerned, since there is absolutely no use in trying to act rational at such a fragile time as this.

N O T E S: ....

....

....

....

....

....

THIRD TRIMESTER

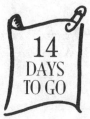

Sometime in the next few weeks, you will
ask yourself, "If the species has relied on
breast-feeding for survival all these millennia,
why is it so hard to learn?" You would think
nothing would be more natural than putting a baby
to your breast and having it feed until satisfied,
but that seldom happens. Instead, the mommy
and the baby both often end up in tears before
a successful "docking maneuver," because latching
on is more complex than a lunar landing.

N O T E S : ....
....
....
....
....
....

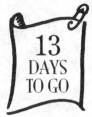

13
DAYS
TO GO

Brand-new babies do not look like the kids in the diaper commercials. Newborns usually look skinny and much smaller than you imagined a human being could be. They also sometimes have downy fur on their shoulders and back. (Don't worry, this disappears soon and remains dormant until the baby turns into a middle-aged man who insists on wearing a muscle T-shirt.) New babies often have complexion problems of their own. Little white zits can cluster around the nose and chin. Don't fuss over these minor imperfections...the world will still recognize that your precious one is just as beautiful as you and Daddy think it is.

N O T E S: ....
....
....
....
....
....

THIRD TRIMESTER

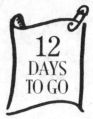

12
DAYS
TO GO

Trust me when I tell you
NURSING DOES NOT PROTECT YOU
FROM GETTING PREGNANT!!!
If you lose your mind and have sex as soon as a
few days after delivery, you can conceive again.
You must use birth control unless you find the idea
of what are known as "Irish twins" appealing.
If you nurse, you will be advised to choose some
form of birth control other than the traditional
pill, probably one with reduced estrogen.

NOTES: ....
....
....
....
....
....

THIRD TRIMESTER

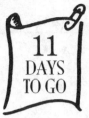

11 DAYS TO GO

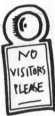

NO VISITORS PLEASE

Get ready for company because new babies draw visitors like a magnet. You are entitled to request no visitors for the first week or two, but after that, people are going to think you are hiding something from them.

Do not feel obligated to clean the house for guests, nor are you expected to offer anything more than a glass of tap water... no matter what your mother says.

N O T E S: ....

....

....

....

....

....

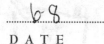

68

D A T E

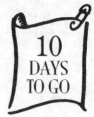

10
DAYS
TO GO

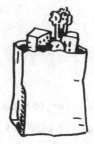

Make sure that you have enough groceries
to last for a couple of weeks.
Sure, you can ask someone to pick up
milk or fruit for you while you're housebound,
but you won't want to reach for toilet paper,
sanitary pads or diapers in the middle
of the night only to find you have run out.

N O T E S: ....
....
....
....
....
....

THIRD TRIMESTER

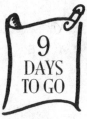

9
DAYS
TO GO

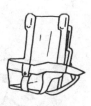

If you haven't already gotten your infant car seat, get it today. If you already have it, spend some time before the baby comes reading the directions. Use a teddy bear as your surrogate baby to practice putting the harness over its wobbly head and releasing the infant carrier from the base that is fastened to the car with a seat belt. The time to learn these maneuvers, which are harder than they look to the uninitiated, is now—not when the baby is crying and you are approaching hysteria.

Remember,
INFANT CAR SEATS MUST FACE THE
REAR OF THE CAR.

N O T E S:...
....
....
....
....
....

THIRD TRIMESTER

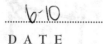
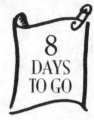

8
DAYS
TO GO

If you don't already have a telephone calling card, get one now. You can buy them in specific credit amounts of $10 or $25 or whatever and use them until you've yakked to their maximum. This is really more a gift for your husband so that he won't have to come to the hospital with pockets jingling full of change for the pay phones. He will have a lot of calls to make when the baby is born, and he might not want to use the phone in your room, either because you're sleeping or because it can't make calls outside the immediate area.

N O T E S: ....

....

....

....

....

....

THIRD TRIMESTER

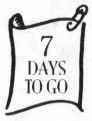

7
DAYS
TO GO

Understand right now that the only way to know for certain that you're in labor is for someone, preferably someone medically trained, to look inside you and see if you're opening up. That means that you are not expected to be able to make that determination yourself. Never, ever, ever be embarrassed if you go to the hospital or call your doctor only to be told that you still have some more waiting to do. You deserve extra attention right now, whether the baby is coming out or not. We promise, no one will be mad at you if you get fooled by those nasty old Braxton Hicks contractions, because they fool nearly everyone.

N O T E S: ....
....
....
....
....
....

THIRD TRIMESTER

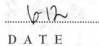

...6.12...

DATE

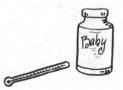

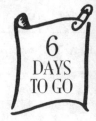

6 DAYS TO GO

Make sure that you have infant acetaminophen (a.k.a. baby Tylenol) and an infant thermometer in the house before you bring the baby home from the hospital. These two things are more important than almost any other baby paraphernalia because you will want to know if your little one has a temperature and be able to bring it down.

Rectal thermometers are the traditional approach (approach, get it?), but they can be terrifying to a new mom. If you simply can't buy one of those new electronic ear thermometers right now, and no one has given you one as an incredibly generous gift, insist that a nurse teach you how to take a rectal temperature before you leave the hospital.

N O T E S : ....
....
....
....
....
....

..6-13...

T E

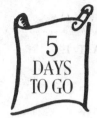

5
DAYS
TO GO

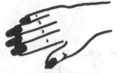

If you have been enjoying the long, strong
ingernails of pregnancy for the last nine (ten)
months, you might want to consider getting a
ensible mommy manicure now. Most of us feel
like we are all thumbs when taking care of
ewborns anyway, and when those thumbs have
ggers on their tips, you risk scratching or poking
e baby. Cut them down to fingertip length and
just put a coat of sheer polish on them since
you won't have time to maintain those
Joan Crawford talons anymore.

N O T E S: ....
....
....
....
....
....

THIRD TRIMESTER

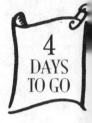

4
DAYS
TO GO

While this is not a La Leche League ad, and
we don't ultimately have the right to dictate
whether you should nurse or not, here is one
thing to consider: Nursing forces us to cut out the
meaningless business of our lives and pay attention
to the baby and ourselves. One of our greatest
mistakes as mothers these days is to rush our
recovery from pregnancy and childbirth. Nursing
can force us overachievers to prioritize our lives
properly to make room for the addition to the
family, rather than darting off to gym classes or
throwing ourselves back into our careers.

N O T E S: ....
....
....
....
....
....

THIRD TRIMESTER

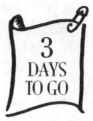

3
DAYS
TO GO

Here's the Ultimate Girlfriends Tip:
The minute you enter the hospital
start asking for an <u>epidural</u> (a combination
of drugs released into the fluid surrounding
your spinal cord through a needle, by an
anesthesiologist, in your lower back) and continue
until you receive one. Labor is not a contest,
you don't win anything by going pain-free
and if you think you want to go au naturel,
talk to me afterward.

NOTES:...
....
....
....
....
....

THIRD TRIMESTER

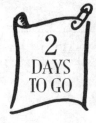

2 DAYS TO GO

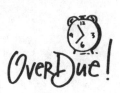

OverDue!

Has your due date come and gone without incident? Don't be too disappointed...
it really is a toss of the coin, since half of the pregnant population will deliver "early" and the other half will deliver "late."

Here's a suggestion: Beg your husband to have passionate, penetrating sex with you tonight. His semen has oxytocin in it, the chemical that brings on contractions. Even if you don't go into labor, you'll have killed some time in a pleasant fashion.

NOTES: ....
....
....
....
....
....

THIRD TRIMESTER

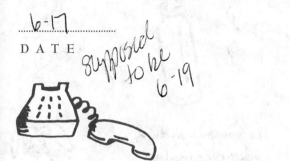

6-17
DATE

supposed to be 6-19

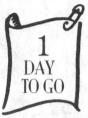

1 DAY TO GO

Still no baby? Trust us when we say, emphatically, that a baby in your belly is easier to take care of than one outside your belly.

Try to rest and, by all means, take your phone off the hook. There is nothing more tedious than having to tell twenty callers a day that no, the baby isn't here yet.

Haul yourself outside for as brisk a walk as you can muster. Walking forces the baby's head gently against your cervix, and it might get things moving in there.

NOTES: ....
....
....
....
....
....

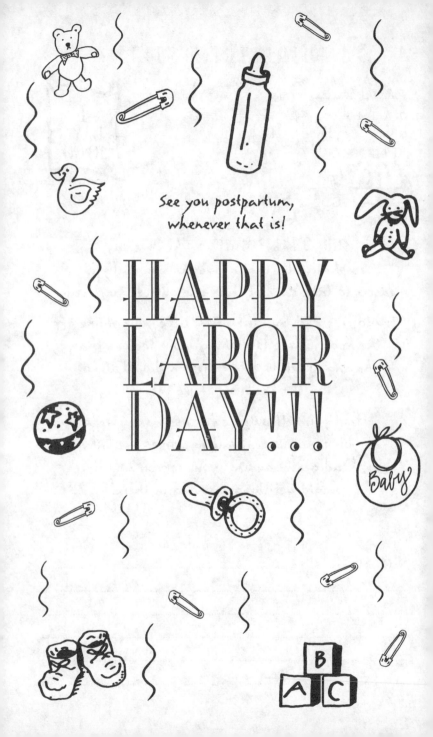

See you postpartum,
whenever that is!

HAPPY
LABOR
DAY!!!...

FOURTH TRIMESTER

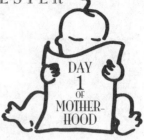

My sister-in-law pushed so hard during delivery
that afterward, the whites of her eyes turned
red. Several of my other Girlfriends noticed
broken capillaries on their cheeks. We've even
met women who bruised under their eyes while
getting that baby out. I just wanted to be the
first to tell you a delivery horror story!

Even if none of these things happens to you, you
will almost certainly find your face swollen and
your eyes puffy a few hours after giving birth.
Ask the nurse for two ice packs, one to put on
your face and one to put between your legs.

NOTES: ....

....

....

....

....

....

FOURTH TRIMESTER

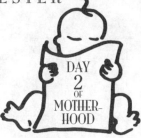

DAY
2
OF
MOTHER-
HOOD

You may have noticed your doctor sucking
fluids out of your baby's nose with a rubber
bulb before the little thing has even gotten all
the way out of your body. Make sure you don't
leave the hospital without one or two of those
nose suckers (feel no guilt because it will show up
somewhere on your hospital bill).

Babies haven't mastered the art of sniffling,
let alone blowing their nose. You can offer a lot
of relief by sticking the bulb in those itsy-bitsy
nostrils, and giving them one good suck.
Babies generally hate it, but us moms love them
almost as much as we love Q-Tips.

N O T E S : ··

··

··

··

··

··

FOURTH TRIMESTER

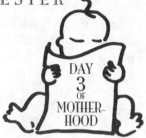

Unbelievable, isn't it? They will
actually trust you enough to send the
baby home in your care. It's ten times
harder to rent a car, even a subcompact!
The people at the hospital know something you
don't: that no one on this planet can care for
this little darling better than its mom.

N O T E S: ....
....
....
....
....
....

FOURTH TRIMESTER

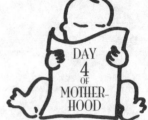

DAY
4
OF
MOTHER-
HOOD

What with episiotomy stitches, hemorrhoids
and the general wear and tear of delivery,
you must be looking forward to your first
bowel movement with the same uncontainable
excitement of someone facing dental surgery.
Suddenly you have pushing flashbacks and
you are filled with dread. Unless you prefer
being full of you-know-what, you
have no choice but to march into that
bathroom and eliminate! Yes, it hurts,
but nothing tears or breaks, contrary to
the vivid sensations.

NOTES:...

....

....

....

....

FOURTH TRIMESTER

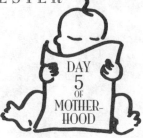

DAY
5
OF
MOTHER-
HOOD

Take a moment to really look at your baby's ears.
Pediatricians maintain that the ear is the last bit
of physical development (along with the lung
membranes) to develop on a fetus, so to really
feel the miracle of this little being, take a look at
the ears...so tiny, and yet there they are with
little lobes, curves and folds. If your baby was
born prematurely, the ears will develop the same,
but it will happen on the outside where you can
watch it. Everyone talks about the relief of
finding ten toes and fingers, but those ears
should at least get equal time.

NOTES:..
....
....
....
....
....

FOURTH TRIMESTER

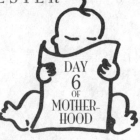
Protecting your baby from germs is critical
in the first few weeks when its immune system
is just warming up, but many mothers can
be obsessed with very little prodding. A pacifier
dropped on the floor doesn't really need to
be destroyed...boiling water would satisfy even
Jonas Salk. A surgical mask on visitors is
rarely called for unless they are spewing phlegm
or have open sores, in which case they shouldn't
be in your neighborhood, let alone holding
your child. Even a good wet kiss from the family
dog will probably do little harm, so keep the dog
and try not to let it drink out of toilets.

NOTES:...

....

....

....

....

....

FOURTH TRIMESTER

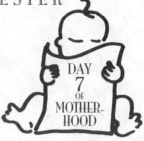

DAY
7
OF
MOTHER-
HOOD

Try lying on your tummy for the first time
in ages. Roll over slowly because your insides
are still sore and out of alignment, and put
a soft pillow under your breasts, which
may be filling with milk.

Doesn't that feel amazing? For the first
time in ages, you can feel the separate
vertebrae in your spine rather than the sensation
that the whole apparatus was fused into
wrought iron months ago.

If you have had a C-section, wait a few more
days, and put a pillow against your incision before
you enjoy this simple pleasure.

NOTES:...
....
....
....
....
....

FOURTH TRIMESTER

DAY
8
OF
MOTHER-
HOOD

If your birth experience was complicated and not what you dreamed it would be, it is very likely that you feel sadness, resentment and maybe even guilt. Some women who ended up with unexpected C-sections still mourn years later that they didn't get the birth they had planned and prepared for. There is a faint inkling that they have failed at something that should have come so naturally to them.

Get over it! You did the right thing, at great sacrifice to yourself, and the truth of that lies in the baby in your arms. But you still need to believe it yourself.

NOTES:

FOURTH TRIMESTER

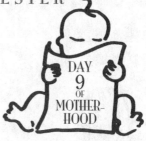

During the week or two following delivery, you are
likely to wake up in the middle of the night so wet
that you swear someone hosed you down. This is
just nature's way of helping you get rid of all the
water you have been retaining. Sleep on towels
until the sauna stage passes, and never sleep in
silky lingerie (as if!) because it just gets cold and
sticky when wet. It's a drag to wake up and find
yourself drowning, but it does lead to weight loss,
and that's what counts.

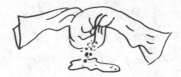

N O T E S: ....
....
....
....
....
....

FOURTH TRIMESTER

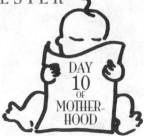

DAY
10
OF
MOTHER-
HOOD

It can be several days, even weeks, before you will be able to stand for more than a minute without having the sensation that your uterus is so heavy that it is going to fall out of your body and land with a splat on the bathroom floor.

Remember that pelvic floor area that you could never identify when you tried out Kegel exercises? Well, guess what? You've found it! See, I wasn't just haranguing you when I told you to keep Kegeling. Start again today, and continue until you are so old that you don't mind wearing a diaper every day.

N O T E S: ....
....
....
....
....
....

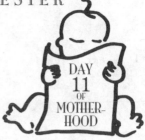

DAY
11
OF
MOTHER-
HOOD

Babies aren't supposed to be tub-bathed until their belly button stumps fall off. I only mention it now because I completely forgot this rule when my fourth baby was born (so much for practice-makes-perfect). As cute as "Baby's First Bath" photos and videos are, there is no good reason to rush into the total body plunge. A wet and sudsy baby is harder to hold on to than a live trout.

Stick with the sponge bathing until your best mommy friend or one of the grandmas come by to spot you. You will also need a third adult in the room, perhaps Daddy, to operate the cameras.

N O T E S : ....
···
···
···
···
···

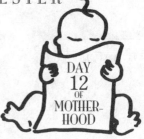

DAY
12
OF
MOTHER-
HOOD

Relax & Nap

Wow, time flies when you're physically
and mentally exhausted. Welcome to the
real world of motherhood. We're here to help
you through the next couple of months,
and our first pearls of wisdom? Hook up
the answering machine
(always screen calls until further notice)
and take a nap.

N O T E S : ....
....
....
....
....
....

FOURTH TRIMESTER

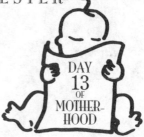

You, too, should avoid tub baths until your
doctor tells you otherwise. Until your cervix closes
up nice and tight again, you run the risk of
introducing bacteria (not to mention bubble bath)
into your uterus. If you need to relieve your
stitches and/or hemorrhoids, go ahead
and sit in three to four inches of hot water
(otherwise known as a sitz bath),
but don't recline (as if you had the time).

N O T E S: ....
....
....
....
....
....

FOURTH TRIMESTER

DAY
14
OF
MOTHER-
HOOD

New moms are often alarmed at the cramps they feel during nursing. They can actually be painful, but this is usually more common with second or third babies.

This sensation is no cause for alarm (at least no more alarming than the countless other excretions, bruises, stitches and herniated tissue that you've already faced). In fact, it is a good thing because it means your uterus is tightening back up to its prepregnancy size of a pear.

N O T E S : ....
....
....
....
....
....

FOURTH TRIMESTER

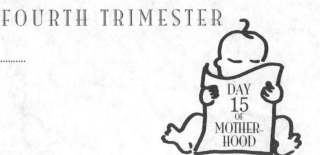

DAY
15
OF
MOTHER-
HOOD

Don't be concerned by the appearance of your
precious baby's belly button. Sure, you were
probably alarmed by how big and dark it looked,
but fear not, because how it looks in the first
few weeks has no bearing on whether it will
ultimately end up an "inny" or an "outy."
Your job at this time is to protect it while the
stump is healing and to keep it clean
(which takes tremendous intestinal fortitude
since we are all afraid to go digging around
in there with our alcohol swabs).

NOTES:...
....
....
....
....
....

FOURTH TRIMESTER

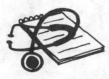

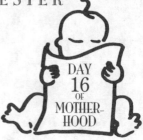

DAY
16
OF
MOTHER-
HOOD

Baby immunizations are unbearably painful; not
for the baby, but for YOU! You know it's time
for that first inoculation, and since you're the
grown-up here, you must take your baby in for its
first brush with a needle. Buck up, Girlfriend,
you'll make that doctor's appointment and you'll
keep it. Most importantly, you will be there holding
your baby in your arms and perhaps offering it
a little nip at the breast for comfort. The little
darling will forget about this travesty by the time
you tuck it back into its car seat, even if you are
still sobbing uncontrollably an hour later.
Mommyhood is not for wimps!

N O T E S: ....

....

....

....

....

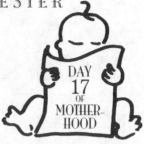

DAY
17
OF
MOTHER-
HOOD

The first couple of weeks (at least) of nursing can be really painful. Our soft nipples will balk at having someone sucking on them constantly. And let's talk about how hard a baby that size can suck! Now's the time for those Lamaze breathing techniques.

By the way, if you had always planned to nurse, don't let this agony be the reason you stop. Try to stick it out one more week. Nursing not only becomes absolutely painless, but the uterine contractions that go along with it actually start feeling vaguely reminiscent of orgasm. Swear to God!

NOTES:..

....

....

....

....

....

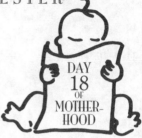

DATE ....

Nipples that are cracked and scabbed will not get better by being rubbed with various nursing creams. Just keep on nursing; the baby won't notice how raggedy you look or feel. The only cure is to break on through to the other side.

When you aren't nursing, take every opportunity to expose your nipples to air. Keep your bra flaps open after you've finished nursing to let them dry. It's really quite a sight for someone who accidentally walks in on you at this time. There is little more you can do for the poor darlings, except perhaps send them on a vacation for two to St. Bart's.

N O T E S: ....

....

....

....

....

....

FOURTH TRIMESTER

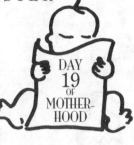

H2O

Have you heard the old folk advice to drink beer to stimulate your milk production? I'm no teetotaler, but this suggestion sounds like a hackneyed excuse (completely understandable, however) to take a nip now and then to dull the latch-on pain. Other than anesthesia, there is little beer contributes that you can't get from a big glass of water. Remember that ultimately, alcohol is a diuretic and will dry you out. There, end of sermon.

N O T E S : ....

....

....

....

....

....

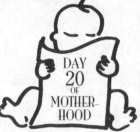

DATE

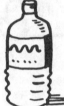

Speaking of water, never sit down to nurse without a huge glass or bottle of water right beside you. As soon as the baby latches on, your mouth will get so dry that your tongue sticks to the roof. Isn't Mother Nature clever to remind you in such a vivid way that the milk factory relies on a steady infusion of water?

Keep bottles of water in all the places where you used to keep antacids. Go to sleep at night with a big glass of ice, so the middle-of-the-night nursing finds you with something remotely cold.

NOTES:

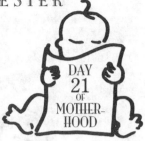

....
DATE

Time to pick up the electric breast
pump you reserved. The places that
rent these pumps are generally staffed
by women who know volumes about babies,
nursing and pumping, so plan to spend
some time with them learning everything
you can. The highlight of the orientation
is when you are shown how to pump
both breasts at the same time! Old Bossy
the Cow has nothing on you, Girlfriend!

N O T E S : ....
....
....
....
....
....

FOURTH TRIMESTER

DAY
22
OF
MOTHER-
HOOD

Is your baby becoming a tyrant? Sure, he fooled
you those first couple of weeks; all he did
was sleep, eat and daintily dirty a diaper now
and then. Now he is crying at all hours,
particularly near dinnertime when you are
most crushingly exhausted, and you are
going crazy with your inability to find the
cause of his misery and cure it.

Guess what, even as we enter the millennium,
no one is really sure what makes babies fussy
or colicky. We only know that this, too,
shall pass—usually by the time the baby is three
months old. Hold on, Girlfriend!

N O T E S: ....
....
....
....
....
....

FOURTH TRIMESTER

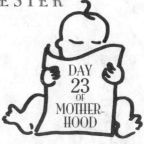

DAY
23
OF
MOTHER-
HOOD

If you are secretly beginning to feel a bit resentful
of your baby's seemingly endless demands, if you
have walked up and down the hall till you've
worn a path in the carpet, nursed so much
that you haven't closed your bra flaps in two
days and if you can't remember the last time
you slept long enough to dream, it's time to reach
out for help. Trust us, since we are undoubtedly
thinking more clearly than you are at this point,
all good moms know when to take a break so
that they can come back to their mothering
tasks with a better outlook and new vitality.
Get a sitter, a husband, or any pair of loving
arms to cover for you, and take a break.

N O T E S: ....

....

....

....

....

....

FOURTH TRIMESTER

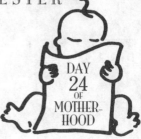

Babies' fingernails are like switchblades, and they can easily scratch the little beauty's face. This presents yet another Mommy Nightmare. It is so easy to cut the nails too short or to nick the baby's soft fingertips. OK, I confess, I cut my son's nails so short that he lost the top layer of his thumb.

1. Cut the nails with baby <u>scissors</u> rather than little <u>clippers</u>.

2. Attempt all manicures when the baby is sleeping. We all know it's impossible to hit a moving target.

3. When all else fails, bite the nails off with your own teeth.

NOTES: ....
....
....
....
....
....

FOURTH TRIMESTER

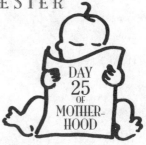

DAY 25 OF MOTHER-HOOD

News flash! Your baby will continue to breathe even when you are not staring at it and willing it to do so. Don't worry, we all have tried to stay awake and vigilant day and night when we brought our tiny little babies home from the hospital, but fatigue eventually strikes down even the most neurotic of us. You must rest. It helps ease some anxiety if you keep the baby in a bassinet beside your bed or if you put the baby monitor in the crib beside the baby so that you can hear every delicious breath it takes.
Now, go lie down.

N O T E S : ....
....
....
....
....
....

DAY
26
OF
MOTHER-
HOOD

If you are nursing, remember to keep your feet up. It's also a good idea to put a cushion or pillow in your lap. The idea here is to bring Mohammed closer to the Mountain. If the baby is up near your nipple, you will have less of a tendency to support her with your arms, a technique that invariably leads to "nursing neck."—a painful stiffness that comes from hours of sitting with your shoulders scrunched while your baby eats.

If anyone asks if you need help, get him to massage your neck and shoulders and bring you an anti-inflammatory.

NOTES:

FOURTH TRIMESTER

DAY
27
OF
MOTHER-
HOOD

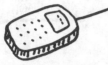

A baby monitor takes some getting used to. First of all, you will be tempted to turn the volume up so high that you will not only hear every whimper, but the sound of the baby's hair growing! Then, when he gives one good cry, you will sustain more hearing damage than a teenager in a mosh pit.

A word of warning: Baby noises are not the only sounds that monitors relay. I know of a father who used the private phone in the nanny's room to set up a tryst while his wife heard the entire illicit conversation over the baby monitor. She has custody, and he has occasional visitation.

N O T E S:..
....
....
....
....
....

FOURTH TRIMESTER

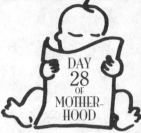

DAY
28
OF
MOTHER-
HOOD

Don't think your husband has become some sort of deviant just because he expresses interest in what your breast milk tastes like. The simple answer is, it tastes rather like coconut milk, and is sort of watery and very sweet.

Chances are, however, he is really more interested in trying out the whole nursing experience. Our advice is, once your nipples have toughened up and no longer hurt, go ahead and give him a little sip. Later, when you find yourself engorged with milk and without a hungry baby or a breast pump nearby, your husband's willingness to suck may be all that stands between you and an explosion.

N O T E S : ....
....
....
....
....
....

FOURTH TRIMESTER

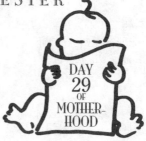

DAY
29
OF
MOTHER-
HOOD

Let's talk about sex again.
Aside from your first postpartum bowel
movement, few things are more terrifying than
the thought of your husband (or even Mel Gibson,
for that matter) penetrating your poor,
traumatized privates. Sure, you sympathize
with his begging and pleading, but don't
make any unnecessary sacrifices. And when
the magic moment arrives, make sure
that you're on top so that you can control
the speed and accuracy.

P.S. See Day 38!

NOTES: ....
....
....
....
....
....

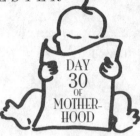

DAY
30
OF
MOTHER-
HOOD

....

D A T E

Nursing in public is a touchy subject. Sooner or later you WILL have to do it, in spite of all plans to the contrary, so here are your options:

You can buy those funny button-front flap shirts that hide your breasts and make it look like you're holding a headless baby. You can cape yourself and the baby with a big receiving blanket, creating a sort of tent for the two of you in the mall or wherever you are. Or, you can simply whip it out, the breast, I mean, and glare at anyone who gives you the hairy eyeball. Pride always fails before a hungry baby's cry.

N O T E S : ....

....

....

....

....

FOURTH TRIMESTER

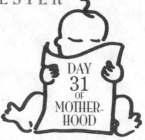

DAY
31
OF
MOTHER-
HOOD

Right about now, you might be quite certain that one child is enough for any family. Who in her right mind would spend another year going through this again, right? There's an old cliché that says, "If it was men who did the birthin', every kid would be an only child."

While this baby's birth may, indeed, complete your family perfectly, most of you will eventually be willing to go back for more. This is not because we women are inherently more courageous than men (although we are), but rather because motherhood causes brain damage and impairs judgment.

N O T E S:...
....
....
....
....
....

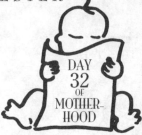

If this is not your first baby, you must be awakening to the fact that no mother in the universe is capable of giving all the time and attention that she thinks each of her children needs and deserves. You are constantly torn between the new baby and your toddler who so clearly misses you.

Try to calm down about it now because it gets worse. Just wait until you go back to work or return to the full responsibilities of running a home. Think of sibling rivalry as a <u>gift</u> to children to hone their social skills and inspire a healthy sense of competition. Whatever you do, don't reveal your frustration to your kids because they have no compassion and will use that information against you later in therapy.

N O T E S: ···

···

···

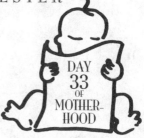

DAY
33
OF
MOTHER-
HOOD

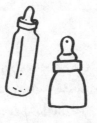

If you are nursing and eventually plan on weaning your child before he can ask for fries with that shake, it's never too early to introduce the bottle. The longer he goes without it, the harder it will be to adapt later. When you do try the bottle, have Daddy give it at the end of the day so you can get some extra hours of uninterrupted sleep and your husband can not only do some bonding, he can put the baby to bed.

NOTES: ....
....
....
....
....
....

DATE
....

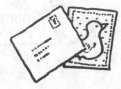

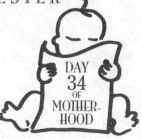

DAY
34
OF
MOTHER-
HOOD

If you have the time and energy, go ahead
and send birth announcements to everyone
you know. Sure, they can be perceived as a
thinly veiled request for gifts, but, hey, no
one is twisting those cynics' arms! This is
the way the Girlfriends see it: The birth of
a baby is a miracle and should be heralded
as such. If you can arrange for the Star of
Bethlehem to shine over your nursery,
why not?

NOTES: ....

....

....

....

....

....

FOURTH TRIMESTER

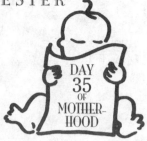

DAY
35
OF
MOTHER-
HOOD

Here's our two cents' worth on the subject
of godparents. If you are of a faith that
has a tradition of naming godparents,
we think you should try to pick blood relatives.
In this transient day, your best friend from
college and your husband's boss may
ultimately not be there for the baby in
the long run. Relatives, no matter how you
feel about them, do tend to stick around.

N O T E S: ....

....

....

....

....

....

FOURTH TRIMESTER

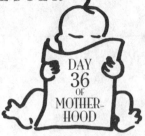

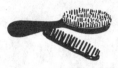

How can we put this to you gently?
Leggings, thick socks with dirty soles, a
giant T-shirt and a bathrobe adorning an
unwashed, unshaved body can actually turn
some men off. Remember, now is not the
time to lose your husband intentionally,
because it's hard to find a replacement
when your breasts are still leaking and you
have fifteen extra pounds glued to you
(and that's BEFORE you pick up the baby!).

N O T E S: ....

....

....

....

....

FOURTH TRIMESTER

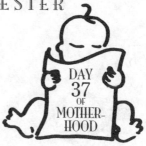

DAY
37
OF
MOTHER-
HOOD

Check on the status of the baby's birth
certificate. You may have sent in the paperwork
from the hospital, but many of us end up
taking home handfuls of paperwork, and
one of those scraps is probably the birth
certificate form. Until you get the official
certificate from the state, you will most
likely have a semiofficial certificate from
the hospital to prove that you have, indeed,
had a baby, not a hallucination.

N O T E S : ....

....

....

....

....

....

FOURTH TRIMESTER

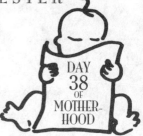

It's about time for your six-week postnatal checkup. Assuming everything down there has healed and shrunk back to a recognizable size, you will be given the green light to have full-tilt sex (as distinguished from satisfying his "needs" through methods that are still illegal in some Southern states).

GIRLFRIENDS UNITE! DO NOT SHARE THE DOCTOR'S "BLESSING" WITH YOUR MATE UNTIL YOU FEEL READY. THE FICTION OF THE SIX-WEEK RECOVERY IS THE RESULT OF A MALE CONSPIRACY!

N O T E S: ....
....
....
....
....
....

FOURTH TRIMESTER

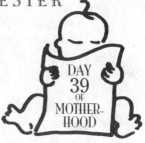

DAY
39
OF
MOTHER-
HOOD

More than half of us new moms have to face
the prospect of going back to work soon, and
we all know how traumatic it feels.
Your attention should be focused on arranging
who will care for your baby while you are at work,
and how to juggle your schedule a bit to
sneak some baby time in. It's a tough
adjustment, since instinct tells us to keep
that baby near us at all times...
but millions of us have done it, and so can you.

N O T E S : ....

....

....

....

....

....

FOURTH TRIMESTER

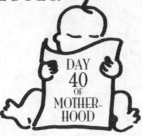

DATE ....

Those of you who only have a six-week maternity leave from work should start preparing for your return now. There are three major concerns:

1. Putting together a presentable wardrobe. Take a look at the things you wore when you were about five months pregnant.

2. Learning to pump your breast milk or beginning to wean your baby onto formula.

3. Trying not to sob any time you think about spending an entire day without your baby. It's like the first day of kindergarten...you cry and mope the entire day, but pretty soon, you realize that seeing all the other kids in school is kind of fun.

NOTES: ....
....
....
....
....
....

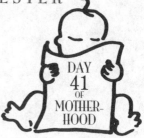

DAY
41
OF
MOTHER-
HOOD

....
DATE

A little tired during that 3 A.M. feeding?
Bring the baby to bed and nurse until
someone falls asleep, husbands not included.
Don't worry, nobody will roll over on the baby
in the middle of the night.
Hard to believe, isn't it?
Check with your doctor, he or she will
assure you that it's perfectly safe.

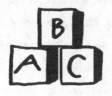

NOTES: ....
....
....
....
....
....

FOURTH TRIMESTER

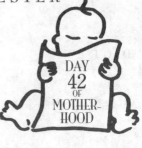

DAY
42
OF
MOTHER-
HOOD

Here you are, back at work, looking pretty good
and having fun seeing the old gang again.
Then all of a sudden it hits you: You have left
your precious baby in the care of someone you
hardly know and pay $300 a week! They can
easily make $10,000 selling your perfect angel on
the black market! What were you thinking?

Here's what you were thinking: You did
your homework and selected the best person
you could find to care for your baby. She is sweet
and nurturing, she has references, and besides,
you've hidden a video camera on the bookshelf
to monitor her every move.

N O T E S: ....

....

....

....

....

....

FOURTH TRIMESTER

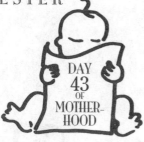

DAY
43
OF
MOTHER-
HOOD

Lots of new moms worry that their baby likes the sitter or housekeeper more than them. Relax, your baby still thinks it is you. Sure, maybe the more experienced care of the sitter (who has done this before) may be more calming to the baby, but that doesn't mean it doesn't love you more than heaven and earth. It probably just means that you smell like milk and when you hold the baby, it thinks it's chow time. In a few months, you will have more obvious evidence that you are the center of your baby's universe...like when you have to sneak out of the house to avoid an awful separation scene.

N O T E S: ....

....

....

....

....

....

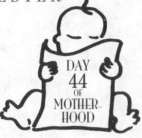

DAY
44
OF
MOTHER-
HOOD

Are three balanced meals a day not on the
top of your priority list? For the baby's sake you
really need your strength, especially if you're a
nursing mom and you're responsible for all her
nutritional needs. Wait until she's toilet-trained
before she exists on a diet of fast food.
But let's not jump ahead.

Now is not the time to be dieting.
Don't you remember? Nine (ten) months up,
nine (ten) months down.

P.S. How are those Kegels
coming along?

NOTES: ....
....
....
....
....
....

FOURTH TRIMESTER

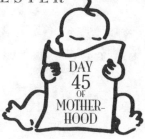

DAY
45
OF
MOTHER-
HOOD

Is your mate feeling left out?
This is a time when it is particularly
difficult to drag your attention from your
enchanting little baby to focus on bathing
yourself, let alone noticing your poor husband.
Try to remember that he used to be
your baby and now he feels like an orphan,
so a little petulance is understandable...
not necessarily curable, but understandable.

N O T E S : ....

....

....

....

....

....

FOURTH TRIMESTER

DAY
46
OF
MOTHER-
HOOD

Start asking around for baby-sitters. I know
the thought of leaving your precious child with
a gum-snapping Lollapalooza fanatic sounds
unthinkable, but there will come a time when
you and your husband will want to get out for
at least the first half of a movie, and it is
imperative that you learn to trust someone
(well, trust may be too strong a word) or
take a chance on someone besides yourself
being able to care for your child.

Good luck. Our prayers are with you.

N O T E S: ....
....
....
....
....
....

FOURTH TRIMESTER

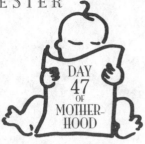

DAY
47
OF
MOTHER-
HOOD

Ready for the big date? Is it about time to
resume "full marital relations" with your mate?
Keep two words in mind: inebriate and lubricate.
A glass of red wine (think goblet-size) does
wonders to relax you and make you feel amorous.
It also helps you forget your terror that your
vagina is going to be ripped to shreds. You will
need the lubrication because you will be dry, dry,
dry down there, no matter how aroused you feel.
Other than that, remind your husband to be gentle
and proceed more slowly than his horniness would
have him go. You'll have fun, even if your orgasm
machine is still out of whack.

NOTES:...
....
....
....
....
....

FOURTH TRIMESTER

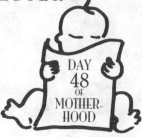

DAY
48
OF
MOTHER-
HOOD

You may already have discovered accidentally what
we're going to tell you now. The loud, droning
sound of certain appliances, such as vacuums,
blenders and blow-dryers, puts lots of babies right
to sleep. When you have some steam to blow or
the baby just won't stop howling, consider putting
the baby in a front pack and vacuuming the house.
Feel free to yell or sing because you just blend in
with the noise. The baby will be snoozing.

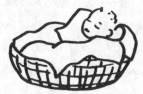

N O T E S: ....
....
....
....
....
....

FOURTH TRIMESTER

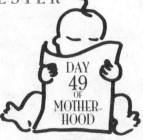

DAY
49
OF
MOTHER-
HOOD

Remember how we told you to
make good use of your obstetrician,
with questions and phone calls?
Well, the same holds true for your pediatrician.
If you're not happy with the practice then move on.
There are no rules that you have to stick it
out with that doctor. The only one you have to
stick it out with is your baby.

N O T E S : ....
....
....
....
....
....

DATE

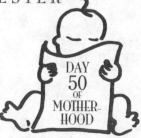

DAY
50
OF
MOTHER-
HOOD

If you are working outside the home
and the baby is not with you, try not
to get into too many conversations about
your little angel. The more vividly and
lovingly you describe him or her, the
more apt you are to feel a longing.
The more longing you feel, the greater
the chance that your letdown reflex
will occur and you will look like an
also-ran in a wet T-shirt contest.

NOTES: ....
....
....
....
....
....

DAY
51
OF
MOTHER-
HOOD

It's time to learn the motherly art of the
"little white lie." Our society and especially
our employers just don't seem to understand
the importance of being there for the critical
life passages of our babies. Sure, you can be
honest and tell everyone that you are leaving
work early, with that important deal
incomplete, because your baby is getting a shot,
but you won't be respected for it. You must create
a non-maternal excuse, such as a sales call
or a meeting outside the office.

NOTES:..
....
....
....
....
....

FOURTH TRIMESTER

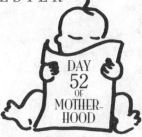

We all know that solitary confinement is
one of the highest forms of punishment
in our penal system. Well, add a crying baby to
that and you have motherhood on a really bad
day. Isolation can be a real problem for new
mommies. Rather than attack your husband each
evening, starving for conversation, pack up the
baby every day and get out of the house.
That's what "mommy and me" groups are for.

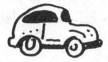

N O T E S: ··

··

··

··

··

FOURTH TRIMESTER

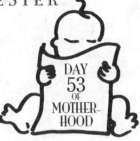

DAY
53
OF
MOTHER-
HOOD

Postpartum depression is real and probably touches all of us new moms to varying degrees, whether we recognize it or not. It is not a sign of failure, nor is it imagined. It is also not a silly little case of tears a couple of days after giving birth, as some books would have you believe. It is the lethal combination of hormonal havoc, exhaustion, isolation and irrevocable change. If you think you have it, call your o.b. today, because you can be helped.

NOTES:..
....
....
....
....
....

FOURTH TRIMESTER

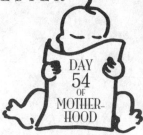

DAY
54
OF
MOTHER-
HOOD

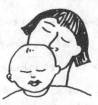

Don't you love the smell of your baby?
Do you know that a study was done where
brand-new moms were blindfolded and
asked to pick out their baby from a group
of several newborns based only on smell?
The mothers were able to pick almost
every time. Isn't nature grand?

N O T E S : ....
....
....
....
....
....

FOURTH TRIMESTER

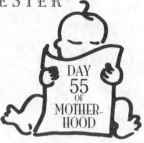

DAY
55
OF
MOTHER-
HOOD

Is this motherhood business a lot
different from what you fantasized
when you were still pregnant? Funny how
that works, isn't it? Those women in
formula commercials singing to their babies
while walking on the beach really piss us off.
That "mom" isn't sleep-deprived,
barfed on, or experiencing postpartum pimples.
She probably isn't even really a mom.

N O T E S : ....

....

....

....

....

....

FOURTH TRIMESTER

DAY
56
OF
MOTHER-
HOOD

Even the most finicky and organized
of us lose all control of our environment
when a new baby comes home to live with us.
You will wonder, as you step over piles
of laundry in every room of the house,
how one tiny baby can require
so much time and work.
Once again, we remind you:
Pregnancy and motherhood are
lessons in surrender.

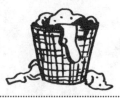

NOTES: ....

....

....

....

....

....

FOURTH TRIMESTER

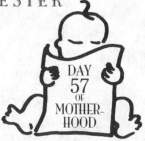

DAY
57
OF
MOTHER-
HOOD

It goes without saying that your husband isn't as good at baby care as you are. You have two choices, as you watch him fling his hand around madly trying to get the diaper tab unstuck from his fingers while keeping the other hand on the baby so he doesn't escape, only to have him pee in his face:

1. You can tell him he's inept and complete the task in your own perfect way, or

2. You can let him struggle through on the assumption that practice makes passable and let him know that he better get the hang of it.

N O T E S:···

··

··

··

··

··

FOURTH TRIMESTER

....
D A T E

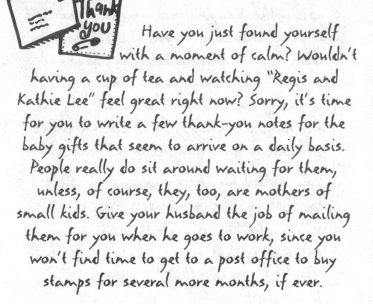

DAY
58
OF
MOTHER-
HOOD

Have you just found yourself with a moment of calm? Wouldn't having a cup of tea and watching "Regis and Kathie Lee" feel great right now? Sorry, it's time for you to write a few thank-you notes for the baby gifts that seem to arrive on a daily basis. People really do sit around waiting for them, unless, of course, they, too, are mothers of small kids. Give your husband the job of mailing them for you when he goes to work, since you won't find time to get to a post office to buy stamps for several more months, if ever.

N O T E S : ....
....
....
....
....
....

FOURTH TRIMESTER

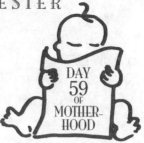

DAY
59
OF
MOTHER-
HOOD

Babies do not give you advance notice
before they roll over for the
first time. That means that you
should expect it to happen at any time.
Never, ever leave the baby on a changing
table or bed for one moment
because that will be the moment it
hurls itself into the wild blue yonder.

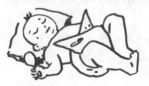

N O T E S: ....

....

....

....

....

....

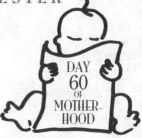

DATE

Mother's intuition is very real and very reliable. Trust your instincts. If you think your baby is feeling sick, it probably is. If you think it hates wearing booties, you're probably right. There is some kind of extraordinary communication between a mother and child (at least until the teen years), and it will guide you in making the right parenting decisions most of the time.

NOTES: ....

....

....

....

....

....

FOURTH TRIMESTER

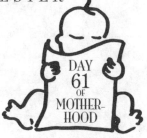

D A T E

Do you secretly believe that no one, particularly
your husband, can properly care for your baby?
Sure, we want the dads to join in and share this
parenting experience, but do we really <u>trust</u> them?
Most of us hover around barking such observations
as "Don't drop her!" or "Watch his neck!" or
"Any fool knows that the picture band goes
on the <u>front</u> of the diaper!"

You're not helping here! Fatigue alone should
soon cure you of this nagging.

N O T E S : ....
....
....
....
....
....

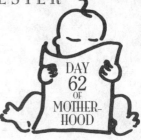

DAY
62
OF
MOTHER-
HOOD

....
DATE

Go ahead and ask your husband the
same question we all feel obliged to ask
when having sex after birth:
"Does it feel the same down there?"
If he is smart, he will lie and tell you
it feels the same, if not better.
Never ask again.

N O T E S: ....
....
....
....
....
....

FOURTH TRIMESTER

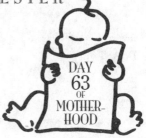

DAY
63
OF
MOTHER-
HOOD

A lazy bladder is a legacy of pregnancy.
Thousands of women who have had vaginal births
cannot sneeze without wetting their pants. Others
say they just can't "hold it" like they used to. You
may find yourself unable to sleep an
entire night without getting up to
use the bathroom. Look at it this
way: A nocturnal stroll gives you a
chance to go in and check on the baby.

NOTES:..
....
....
....
....
....

FOURTH TRIMESTER

DAY
64
OF
MOTHER-
HOOD

If you have a pretty good marriage to begin
with, adding a baby to the mix just makes
it better. Suddenly, you love your mate not
just because he's sweet or cute or sexy...
you love him because he loves your child.
In years to come, you will almost ache with love
for what a good daddy he is and how bonded the
two of you are in your commitment to your
family. Then, again, there will be times that
you have the biggest fights of your life over
differing parenting styles. C'est la vie!

N O T E S: ....
....
....
....
....
....

FOURTH TRIMESTER

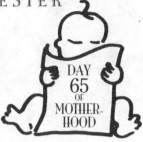

DAY
65
OF
MOTHER-
HOOD

Never wake a sleeping baby.
We know they look so delicious lying there
asleep, their little mouths sleep-sucking,
their little hands in fists under their chins,
but don't pick them up! Feel free to look until
the image is etched into your heart,
but then you must go and rest for a few minutes.
This opportunity will not last forever.

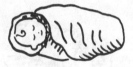

N O T E S :...

....

....

....

....

....

....

D A T E

DAY
66
OF
MOTHER-
HOOD

Baby swings can be emancipation for new
moms. As you well know, babies prefer
gentle movement to being still, but that movement
does not necessarily have to be provided
exclusively by you. Borrow or buy a swing and
set it up near you. You may have as long
as an hour to make dinner, take a
shower or watch *The Rosie O'Donnell Show*
without a baby in your arms.

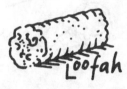

Loofah

N O T E S: ....
....
....
....
....
....

FOURTH TRIMESTER

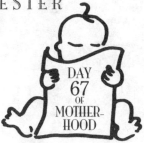

Many mothers feel such love and devotion for their baby that they live in a constant state of terror. They know one thing for certain...if something were to happen to their baby, they would never survive it.

First, let's rush to remind ourselves that our children will be fine and still around long after they have lost most of their charm. Then, let's feel the awe at the bond between mothers and babies. It's a love so fierce it can literally make your heart hurt. Welcome to the Order of the Perpetually Vulnerable.

N O T E S:...
....
....
....
....
....

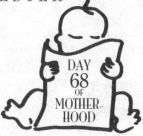

DAY
68
OF
MOTHER-
HOOD

....
D A T E

If you are still nursing, you may doubt this information, but it will ring true eventually: The breasts of women who have birthed babies will never regain their prepregnancy fullness and firmness. Think <u>National Geographic</u> for a visual cue. Anyone who tells you different is either a fluke of nature or neglecting to mention a certain plastic surgeon in her life.

N O T E S: ....

....

....

....

....

....

FOURTH TRIMESTER

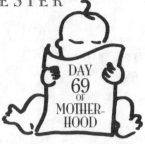

DAY
69
OF
MOTHER-
HOOD

It's never too early to learn not to waste
time comparing your child's development
with others. Everybody knows someone
whose baby is a month younger than yours
and already sleeps through the night. Later, it will
be the baby who walks before yours does or
is potty-trained in one day at eighteen months.
Ignore it all. Someday, all of these kids will be
working for your late-blooming genius.

N O T E S : ....
....
....
....
....
....

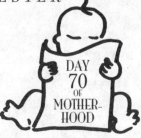

DAY
70
OF
MOTHER-
HOOD

....

D A T E

Are you nursing? Have you had sex yet
that was truly arousing, not just merciful?
Then you must be familiar with the
"car wash" phenomenon. Women with sensitive
"letdown" reflexes have been known to
climax and spray milk simultaneously.
Consider putting your nursing bra back on
after the foreplay, and use extra pads.

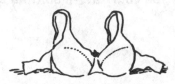

N O T E S : ....

....

....

....

....

....

FOURTH TRIMESTER

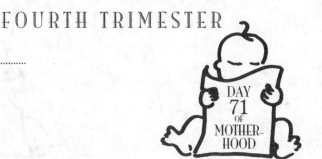

DAY
71
OF
MOTHER-
HOOD

New mothers often become environmental
activists. They didn't mind living in air
pollution themselves, but they put up a
holler if their baby's precious lungs are
vulnerable. Anyone lighting up a cigar risks
personal injury, and I don't mean
from the tobacco.

N O T E S :..
....
....
....
....
....

FOURTH TRIMESTER

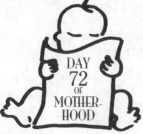

If you've already fallen behind or given up
on the baby book, don't worry.
Look at it this way: Odds are you'll never
have time to do it for a sibling
(easy for us to plan ahead), so it's not
fair to do it for the firstborn. And if this
is an only child, he will have no frame
of reference. Are we Girlfriends good at
rationalization or what?

N O T E S: ....

....

....

....

....

....

FOURTH TRIMESTER

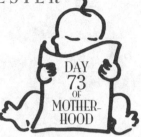

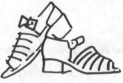

If your feet got bigger during your
pregnancy, and we're pretty sure they did,
then about now you must be wondering
when they are going to shrink back to their
normal size. You can stop wondering because this
bigger foot <u>is</u> your new normal size.

Look at the bright side...you have a great
excuse to buy new shoes, and this foot
growth usually happens only once in your
reproductive life, even if you have ten more kids.

N O T E S: ....

....

....

....

....

....

DATE

DAY
74
OF
MOTHER-
HOOD

Now that you and your husband are officially "grown up" (by virtue of being someone's parents), it is time to draft a will. If you don't legally state how you would want things to go if something were to happen to you, the state decides. Horrifying concept, isn't it? About the state, I mean.

Even if you have no great wealth to provide for, you must decide who would take care of your child if neither of you could. OK, stop crying. We don't have to talk about it any more today.

NOTES: ....
....
....
....
....
....

FOURTH TRIMESTER

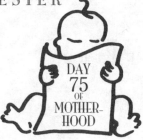

DAY
75
OF
MOTHER-
HOOD

You are not lacking in maternal instinct
if the presence of other children close to
your precious baby drives you crazy.
You are completely correct in your opinion
that children are perpetually moving,
bacteria-producing threats to your infant's
well-being, and that includes
your own older children.

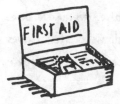

N O T E S: ....
....
....
....
....
....

DAY
76
OF
MOTHER-
HOOD

If you have gotten sick since the baby
was born, then you know the deep,
dark secret: If you're a mommy, it is a
LUXURY to be too sick to get out of bed.
In your child-free days, a silly little chest
cold could be enough to send you straight for the
couch, wrapped in a blanket. Now you have
to be bleeding profusely before someone
steps in and takes over for you. Unfortunately,
the same phenomenon does not apply to
your husband, who still turns into a baby as
soon as his temperature soars to 99 degrees.

N O T E S:...
....
....
....
....
....

FOURTH TRIMESTER

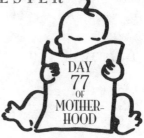

DAY
77
OF
MOTHER-
HOOD

Do not join a gym yet! Sure, you're sick
and tired of looking chubby and flabby,
but your salvation does not lie in a program
of muscle building. If you are still fat and you add
muscle underneath, you will look twice as fat!
Walk, walk, walk, up to sixty minutes a day
if you can, until you are within five pounds of your
desired weight, and then you can start going
for the six-pack stomach and the sinewy triceps.
(We can dream, can't we?)

N O T E S:..
....
....
....
....
....

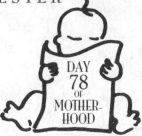

DATE

DAY
78
OF
MOTHER-
HOOD

You will have noticed early on
in your pregnancy that your nipples
got larger and darker; and especially
if you're nursing, they still are.
About nine (ten) months postpartum,
they will return to their former
circumference, but they probably
will not go back to their old color.

NOTES: ....

....

....

....

....

....

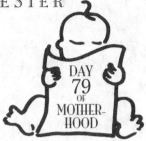

DAY
79
OF
MOTHER-
HOOD

....
D A T E

Forgetfulness is a hallmark of
motherhood. You can't count the number of times
you've walked into a room to do something and
entirely forgotten what it was you intended to do.
It happens in grocery stores, at work, in malls,
everywhere. Get used to it...
it just gets worse until it is replaced by senility.

N O T E S: ....
....
....
....
....
....

FOURTH TRIMESTER

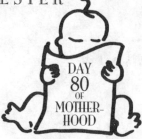

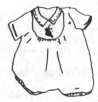

Stop wasting your time with
presoaks and scrubbing. Baby "erp"
stains their shirts, especially if they
drink formulas. You can recycle
much of your infant's wardrobe with
subsequent children, but those shirts
and nightgowns just might be too yellow.

NOTES:..
....
....
....
....
....

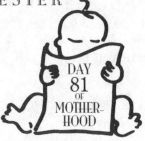

Some mothers, usually women without
full-time jobs or other children, believe in
teaching newborns language through the use
of flash cards...or worse, it is the father who is
eager to give his baby a head start and he
suggests that "since you have some extra time
on your hands," you should devote it to developing
the mind of your baby, since you are both
convinced she's a genius anyway.

It all sounds like a headache to us Girlfriends, for
both you and your barely focusing baby.
Skip the cards and take up singing to your
baby...it's less pressure.

N O T E S: ....

....

....

....

....

FOURTH TRIMESTER

DAY
82
OF
MOTHER-
HOOD

We spend most of our lives grateful that our mothers don't live with us, or even near us. But, when you become a mother, that dynamic can change. Your husband is probably back at work, and there you are, alone with a baby.

Reach out. You are not expected to do this all alone. If your mother-in-law hints that she might like to visit, send her a ticket (round-trip) immediately, even if you think she doesn't approve of you. As the mother of her beloved grandchild, she will do anything for the baby. Ask for advice, accept it and know that she loves the baby nearly as much as you do.

N O T E S : ....

....

.... *Ticket*

....

....

....

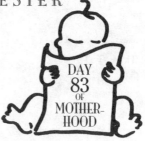

Meet other mommies. Look into
parent-baby groups at your church,
community center or among your Girlfriends.
Not only does misery love company,
but a forum for questions and concerns,
as well as heaps of reassurance,
goes miles in keeping a new mother sane.
This is too big a job for you to do alone.

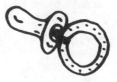

NOTES: ....

....

....

....

....

....

FOURTH TRIMESTER

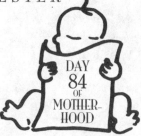

DAY
84
OF
MOTHER-
HOOD

I don't care whether you're a coal miner,
a brain surgeon or a probation officer,
there is no job harder than being a mother.
Other jobs allow you to sleep occasionally,
they don't dictate what you can eat or drink,
they don't expect you to offer your body
as nourishment—and at other jobs,
people occasionally say "thank you."

N O T E S: ....

....

....

....

....

....

FOURTH TRIMESTER

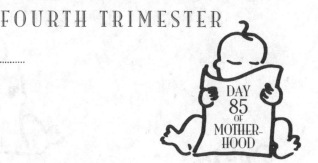

DAY
85
OF
MOTHER-
HOOD

Are you afraid you might be going bald and
are freaking out? Calm down, Girlfriend,
it happens to the best of us. One day, when
you are shampooing, you notice hunks of
hair coming out, and you begin to sweat,
even though you are already wet.

When pregnant, your normal hair loss of
a few strands a day stops, but, after the birth,
your scalp releases the hair that it held on to
during pregnancy. It can look quite dramatic, but
don't reach for the Minoxidil yet, because it will
calm down long before other people notice a thing.

N O T E S : ....

....

....

....

....

FOURTH TRIMESTER

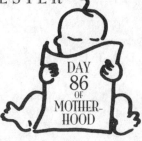

DAY
86
OF
MOTHER-
HOOD

....

D A T E

Relax & Nap

"Nine (ten) months up,
nine (ten) months down"
is the Girlfriends' motto about pregnancy
weight gain and loss. Please do not start
fretting now because you still have chubby
thighs and a belly with the consistency of
bread dough. You are not supposed to be thin
yet; you are still pregnant, remember?
The baby isn't in your tummy anymore,
but your body is still in an altered state.

Now, calm down and take a nap.

N O T E S: ....
....
....
....
....
....

FOURTH TRIMESTER

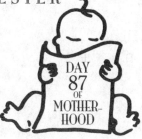

Motherhood is a marathon, not a sprint.
The key to finishing this race is conserving energy
and setting a reasonable pace. Now is not the
time to learn Chinese cooking or repaint the
garage doors, even if those silly books and
magazines insist all homemakers do it.

Consider yourself eminently productive if you
and your baby have eaten, been bathed,
put on clean clothes and watched <u>Oprah</u>.
Anything more is ludicrous.

N O T E S : ....
....
....
....
....
....

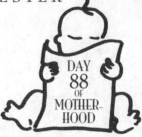

DATE

....

Take this little bit of Girlfriend wisdom and carry it with you for the rest of your mothering days: You will never really know how good a mother you have been. Even when you have a promising college graduate sending you thrilling and literate letters from the Peace Corps, you may have another child of your womb, who was raised with all your love and care, who collects roadkill and puts it in the freezer. No matter what, they will continue to change inexplicably. As hard as it is to believe, studies have proved you will love them anyway.

NOTES: ....

....

....

....

....

....

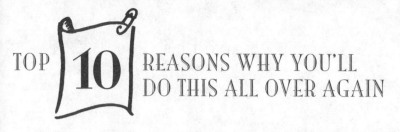

TOP **10** REASONS WHY YOU'LL DO THIS ALL OVER AGAIN

10. MOMMIES' ALZHEIMER'S...YOU'VE ALREADY FORGOTTEN ALL THE WORST PARTS.

9. YOU'VE SPENT SO MUCH MONEY ON BABY STUFF, YOU NEED SEVERAL BABIES TO JUSTIFY THE EXPENSE.

8. IT'S A GOOD EXCUSE FOR NOT LOSING THOSE LAST FIFTEEN POUNDS.

7. YOU NEED ANOTHER BABY TO KEEP ALL THE GRANDPARENTS FROM FIGHTING OVER THE ONE YOU HAVE.

6. YOU ACTUALLY BELIEVED THAT NURSING MOTHERS CAN'T GET PREGNANT.

5. YOU ARE SO TIRED THAT YOU COULDN'T REMEMBER IF YOU INSERTED YOUR DIAPHRAGM OR JUST CONSIDERED IT A GOOD IDEA.

4. YOU WANT THOSE GIGANTIC TITTIES BACK.

3. YOU KNOW WHAT THEY SAY ABOUT AN ONLY CHILD....

2. AN ADDICTION TO THE INTOXICATING SMELL FOUND IN THAT FOLD OF SKIN RIGHT WHERE THE BABY'S FAT LITTLE NECK MEETS ITS FAT LITTLE SHOULDER.

1. WINE.

NOTES

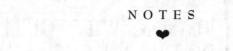

NOTES

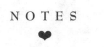

NOTES